New Hope
for
Relief
from Pain

NEW HOPE
FOR
RELIEF
FROM PAIN

by David J. LaFia, M.D.

HAWTHORN BOOKS, INC.
PUBLISHERS/*New York*

For PETER J. STEINCROHN, M.D.,
dedicated physician and friend, who after twenty-five years
at the bedside helping thousands find relief from pain and
suffering turned to medical writing to help millions through
his daily newspaper column, "Stop Killing Yourself," and his
wise books.

He preaches patience that never knew pain.

—*Proverbs*

1814356

We must all die. But that I can save him from days of torture, that is what I feel as my great and ever new privilege. Pain is a more terrible lord of mankind than even death himself.

—*Albert Schweitzer*

The Fellowship of those who bear the Mark of Pain. Who are the members of this Fellowship? Those who have learnt by experience what physical pain and bodily anguish mean, belong together all the world over; they are united by a secret bond.

—*Albert Schweitzer*

The art of life is the art of avoiding pain.

—*Thomas Jefferson*

CONTENTS

INTRODUCTION

"I'm sorry, but you'll just have to live with it."

This advice, heard by so many who have gone to doctors seeking relief from pain, is no longer valid. There *is* hope for chronic sufferers. Never before has so much work been done by so many different specialists to find new ways to control suffering.

Despite the great advances made in controlling pain, too many victims of chronic disabilities have pulled themselves into "pain holes" because they have been told so many times in the past: "I'm sorry, but you'll just have to live with it. There's nothing we can do to help you."

How desperate these people are for some hope of relief from their constant agony is shown in the way they descended on physicians like wild locusts after honey when the ancient Chinese practice of acupuncture began receiving widespread publicity in the Western world.

"Doctor, can it help *me*?" was the substance of their anxious inquiries. "Can you stick silver needles in my body and stop this constant misery that's driving me crazy?"

The answer to such questions is that acupuncture does work *in many cases*. Doctor J. Corcos, a specialist in arthritis and acupuncture, in an article in the May 1973 issue of *Vogue* magazine, said, "Acupuncture's application to all the chronic diseases which involve constant pain and disability is obvious."

Other physicians who have investigated this ancient method of treating pain have made similar reports. And my own experience with acupuncture has convinced me that their conclusions are sound.

How and why acupuncture works are other questions that have not received satisfactory answers as yet. The great demand for acupuncture as a means of alleviating pain means that we, in the United States, have *not* been able with all our scientific, sophisticated methods and techniques to help *most* of these sufferers of long established pain.

It is part of my work as a neurosurgeon to see and treat a seemingly endless number of patients suffering from chronic pain. As I discuss with them the history of their complaints, most have told me bitter and often heartrending tales of their long search for relief. All too often I've heard them say, "I was told that there was nothing medical science could do for me. I just had to learn to live with my pain."

The trouble is that people cannot learn to live silently and miserably with their pain. They may crawl into what I call pains holes for a while. But sooner or later a newspaper announcement of a new technique, a magazine article about a revolutionary wonder drug, or an enthusiastic report on the pain-killing aspects of acupuncture will set them off on another search for relief. Regardless of how much they respect the integrity and knowledge of their doctors, they cannot in the end accept any diagnosis that requires them to live with their pain. They keep searching, spending millions of dollars collectively on painkillers hawked on TV and radio. They spend more millions following the advice of friends and relatives who "knew someone who had just what you've got," and then pour still more money into current fads like the magic vitamin E that is supposed to cure all ills of the flesh from falling hair to impotence in a ninety-five-year-old man!

Most of these searches for painkillers have been in vain. But this does not mean that the search is hopeless. Quite the contrary. Take a quick, imaginary trip around the world with me, and we can peek in on some of the things that are being done worldwide to relieve pain. In each of these cases pain was relieved, and they were all cases in which any physician would have been justified at one time in telling his patient: "There is nothing medical science can do for you. You'll just have to live with it."

In the first case a team of medical specialists at a famous American clinic is examining a distraught, middle-aged woman who is suffering a constant and excruciating facial pain. The advanced diagnostic techniques can find no organic reason for her trouble. The diagnosis is masked depression, and she is advised to accept psychiatric treatments instead of wasting money on powerful drugs and injections into the nerves of her face.

Halfway around the world a high official in the Communist Chinese government consults his acupuncturist. He complains of a persistent pain in his shoulder. The acupuncturist selects a point between the thumb and index finger—called *Ho Ku*—and skillfully inserts his silver needles. The patient reports that he feels relieved of the pain.

In Paris a patient complains of severe burning sensations in the entire left half of his body. The complaint follows a stroke. The pain is so excruciating that he is at the point of suicide, when he consults Dr. Jean Talairach, one of the pioneers of stereotaxic neurosurgery. In this type of operation, Dr. Talairach, using sophisticated equipment, skillfully places a fine wire electrode into the patient's brain. The area is the right thalamus, a mass of gray matter at the base of the brain that is involved in the transmission of sensations. In effect, the doctor is short-circuiting the pain sensations. The result is a partial relief of the patient's agonizing pain.

In Chicago a patient dying of cancer is doomed to live another six months with unbearable pain in the right hip and leg. His pain is relieved by an operation known as percutaneous cordotomy. The originator of this technique, Dr. Sean Mullan of the University of Chicago, inserts a fine wire electrode into the pain pathway of the patient's spinal cord.

In Montreal, Canada, a patient is dying of breast cancer. The malignancy has spread into her bone, causing excruciating pain that is relieved for a few months by the skillful surgery of Dr. Jules Hardy. Dr. Hardy uses highly advanced techniques such as those the public often sees simulated on TV shows such as "The Bold Ones." We see Dr. Hardy placing fine microinstruments through the patient's nasal cavity to destroy the pituitary gland, the small endocrine gland at the base of the brain whose hormones control growth and metabolism. Thanks to Dr. Hardy's skill, this patient is relieved of pain and is capable of enjoying life for the months remaining to her.

In Seattle, Dr. John Bonica, a world-renowned expert on pain control, reviews the management of a pain problem with his staff at the University of Washington Medical School during the weekly meeting of his pain control group. Joining him are specialists in fields such as general and cancer surgery, psychology and psychiatry, neurosurgery, radiotherapy, and anesthesiology. Dr. Bonica is chairman of the Department of Anesthesiology. He demonstrates to his group how chronic pain can be relieved and studied by skillfully blocking the nerves. It is a technique of which he is a master.

These remarkable examples are some of the things that medical science is doing to help relieve chronic pain. However, there is a lot that a patient can do to help himself. In some cases he can do as much as a doctor can do. The fight against pain is not a doctor's fight alone. The patient must do his or her part as well.

This certainly does not mean that a sufferer can serve as his own doctor; medical diagnosis is too complex ever to become a do-it-yourself job. Similar symptoms can come from widely different ailments, and treatments must be carefully observed. Many of the so-called wonder drugs cause serious side effects that could possibly do more damage to the body than the ailment that they cure. They must be administered under the strictest supervision to avoid such side effects.

But regardless, there is a definite and important place for self-help in the struggle against pain. Self-help means not only what you can do for yourself but also whom to see for help, when to see them, and why.

1

RELIEF
FROM PAIN

Relief from pain. Three simple words that mean everything in the world to anyone who suffers from the chronic misery of headache, backache, or stiff joints and stiff fingers. Is there really such a blessing as relief from long established pains? I think so.

Yes, you can find relief from pain, but not by magic. Never before has so much research been conducted for finding new methods of relieving pain, bringing new hope to all sufferers. But to take advantage of this work, you have to keep up your own spirit while you look for help with an open mind.

Chinese acupuncture is playing a role in this new hope for relief from pain. This ancient and definitely useful art of controlling pain works in some cases, but unfortunately too many miraculous claims have been made. Eventually, I think, acupuncture will take its place as an important member of the pain-controlling team, but it is not a cure-all.

Other techniques are being developed. Neurosurgeons have been busy developing safer methods to relieve the pain of cancer and neuralgia without resorting to open surgery. Equally important, psychologists have been probing man's mind to help him understand and overcome his reactions to pain and suffering. This understanding is extremely important, for a patient's mental attitude toward his troubles is a vital factor in his treatment and in his final recovery. Great psychological strides have been made to help patients accept the reality of suffering and death. This is especially true in cancer patients.

You and I live today in a wonderful era, in which pain is beginning to be controlled. But unlike Aladdin, we cannot summon genies to help us by rubbing magic lamps. We must look for help patiently, and our reward will be relief from endless days and nights of living with pain.

The search is not always easy for either the doctor or the patient. The cause of pain is often difficult to find. And once the cause has been isolated, it may be revealed that there are other contributing factors. As an example of how the source of pain is traced, let me tell you about Olga's back pains, since back pains and headaches seem to be the most common types of suffering known to the human race.

Olga and Her Aching Back

Olga is a thirty-two-year-old mother of three children who were born three years apart. The oldest has just turned thirteen. Olga is an active, bustling redhead with a temper as fiery as the color of her hair. She is physically and psychologically unable to take things easy. She must be doing something every waking minute. In addition to housework and caring for her three children, she has been working as a telephone receptionist, since the failure of her husband's small restaurant put them badly in debt. If it should be necessary to describe her in three words, those words would be: *Rush, rush, rush!*

One Monday morning, Olga was rushing as usual to get her six-year-old to school before she reported to work. As she slid into the front seat of her car, Olga felt a sharp twinge of pain in her lower back. It grew worse as the day progressed, and at work she could barely sit due to the pangs of throbbing pain that were coming from her left sacroiliac region, the area in which the backbone joins the pelvis and a common source of low back pain.

Olga was able to finish the day's work only by taking aspirin and lying down during her lunch break. That night she used heating pads and more aspirin. In addition, her husband, Charlie, helped with a rubdown of Ben-Gay ointment, which they had seen advertised as affording relief from local pains. These home treatments only provided minimal relief from the pain, which had spread from the left sacroiliac region all through her left hip.

The next morning Olga could not get out of bed, and this inability to move about grated on her nerves almost as badly as the pain itself. Her husband took the children to school and then went to work himself. Later in the morning, a combination of her trouble and her fretting along with its accompanying strain put her in such misery that she finally decided that the pain was not going to just go away with a little rest. With help from a neighbor, Olga managed to hobble to a car and was driven to the doctor.

The family physician examined her carefully and completely. At the end he told her, "Olga, you've got an acute lumbosacral sprain."

"What's *that*?" she cried in alarm.

"Nothing to get all that excited about," he said with a soothing smile. "The lumbar region is the loins, and the sacral area is at the base of the spine. Medical terms are selected for their descriptive quality so a doctor in one part of the country can understand another without being confused by colloquialisms. They are sometimes frightening to a layman, I know. But you have no cause for great alarm. It simply means that you have a low back pain."

"*That* sounds better," Olga said, and her relief was obvious. "But what caused it? I wasn't lifting anything. I was just getting in the car when it struck me."

"This part of the back bears a terrific strain. The entire weight of the upper part of the body bears down upon it. It is easy to injure, and sacroiliac troubles are very common. There is no way to tell readily what the exact source of your trouble is. We'll have to continue making tests. But in the meantime we'll assume that it is an acute sprain and begin treating that."

"What is the treatment?" she asked, wincing as she tried to move to a more comfortable position in her chair.

"You need daily treatments of hot packs and ultrasound waves to relax the strain and tension in your lower back muscles," the family doctor replied. "Can you manage to get over here each day?"

Olga underwent this conservative treatment for a week. Her pain was as great as ever. Disappointed and near despair, she told her doctor: "This isn't helping me at all! What do I do now?"

"You'll have to go to the hospital for a couple of weeks of complete bed rest, pelvic traction, and some additional tests," he replied.

"Hospital!" she said uneasily. "I—I don't know."

Her fright was obvious, but by now the pain had spread into her left leg. She had heard so many stories from friends and neighbors about people becoming paralyzed from bad backs. She had even been advised by some to never let any doctor operate on her back. She was sick with pain and already feeling like a permanent cripple. She had never had a confining sickness before, and her inability to rush around as she always had was making her condition worse.

Her husband, badly worried about his wife's failure to respond to treatment, talked to the family doctor.

"So there's something wrong with her back," he said, nervously puffing on a cigarette. "Isn't there some kind of back specialist who knows about these things?"

The family doctor replied, "Not really. The back falls into the realm of many types of specialists. That's why I want Olga in the hospital. I intend to call in an orthopedic specialist and, if necessary, a nerve man as well. When I do, the first thing they'll ask me is what *isn't* wrong with her. They will have expected me to have made all the necessary tests to determine that Olga's trouble is not something removed from their specialty."

"But if it's her back——" Charlie began.

"It's her back alright, but *what* in her back? A sprained muscle? A slipped disc? A cancerous condition? Or maybe it isn't connected with the spine or bones at all. It could even be a kidney stone. That's why I must have her in the hospital. We must make tests. If we can't find the exact cause, we will be miles ahead just by eliminating possible causes that aren't the source of the trouble."

Charlie was silent for a moment, sitting with bowed head. Then he said, "This sounds like something big, doc. Something that will take time and money."

"And it will take a lot more time and even more money if she doesn't start cooperating in her treatment. The best thing for her right now is to get off her feet. She has got to give her back some rest. And don't try to tell me that she stays in bed!"

"Well," Charlie said lamely, "I try to get her to keep off her feet, but you know how she is. She'll lie down for a while, and then she's trying to get up again. She's just not the be-still type."

"I know," the doctor replied. "But do what you can to make her take things easy. If she's not better in a few more days, then she must go to the hospital for complete rest, traction, and examinations to rule out the possibilities of diseases of the kidneys and spine."

Charlie got up. "I'll do the best I can to make her stay in

bed," he said. "As for the hospital, I'll have to let you know. It sounds pretty expensive. Not that I mind the expense if it will help her. It's just that I'm so far in the hole now that I'm not sure I can get any more credit."

Olga still refused to face the inevitable. She insisted that Charlie take her to a chiropractor. A neighbor had told her that medical doctors did not know much about the human back. A chiropractor, whose specialty was manipulating and adjusting the spine, the neighbor insisted, was just what she needed.

The chiropractor made a complete X ray of Olga's spine and then gave her a manipulation. For a few hours after the first treatment Olga felt better. She and Charlie were elated, thinking she was at last on the way to a cure. But that night her pain was as bad as ever.

The fact that her pain had been lessened for a short time greatly encouraged her. She went back for six more treatments. During this time her back pain definitely improved, but she continued to have throbbing pain in her left leg.

The chiropractor then told her that he could not help her anymore. "I've been able to lessen your back pain," he told her. "But this throbbing pain running down into your left legs indicates sciatica. This is usually caused by a piece of ruptured disc from the spine pressing on the sciatic nerve. A chiropractor can't help you with that. You may need a neurosurgeon—a specialist in nerves."

Olga and Charlie expressed their appreciation for the chiropractor's honesty in not continuing treatments after he was convinced that they could no longer help her. But they were beside themselves with worry. Then Charlie called their family doctor to make arrangements for Olga to enter the hospital for the examinations that the doctor had insisted upon earlier.

Complete examinations were made, including X rays of her spine and kidneys. Then special consultations were arranged with an orthopedic specialist and a neurosurgeon, bringing together consulting surgeons experienced in both the deformities of bones and joints and the ills of the nervous system. This is the point at which I entered the case.

As a neurosurgeon, my diagnosis was nerve root pressure from a herniated disc. The orthopedic surgeon concurred in this diagnosis. The diagnosis proved correct. It may seem to the uninitiated that pinpointing Olga's difficulty came quickly and that this implies criticism of the doctor who had treated her initially. This is certainly not true. The quick diagnosis was possible because of the preliminary work that was done by Olga's family doctor. His tests and examinations had already eliminated many of the possible sources of trouble in her case. This allowed the two specialists to concentrate on their own fields.

It was explained to the patient that nerve pressure from a herniated disc is not nearly as bad as it sounds. The spine is composed of a series of bones separated from each other by pads or discs of cartilage. These discs serve as pads between the individual bones of the spine. Sometimes these discs are herniated or ruptured out of their proper seat between the bones. The spine also consists of a network of nerves leading to the brain. In Olga's case the herniated disc had pressed against a nerve. This was the source of her excruciating pain. The fact that pain developed in one of her legs indicated that this was the sciatic nerve, which passes down the back of the thigh.

Olga's treatment began with some injections of Novocain into her sore back muscles. This temporarily relieved pain and reduced tension that was putting additional pressure on the source of the trouble. A special corset was then ordered for her to wear.

In the physical therapy department Olga was taught the proper way to sit, stand, and walk. Again the objective was to relieve unnecessary strain on her injured back. She was also taught isometric exercises to increase her body tone. Isometrics were once described as exerciseless exercises. They don't require a lot of violent movement like so many exercises. An example is to press down hard with the fist of one hand into the palm of the other hand, which is pressing upward just as hard. Another isometric is to stand in an open doorway and press the palms of the hand against opposite facings. These and similar exercises make muscles work against each other very effectively without a lot of movement. Thus, they are ideal for maintaining body tone in cases like Olga's, where excessive movement is to be avoided.

At home, a firm mattress and a one-inch-thick board under the mattress were put on her bed. This was to hold her body straight and prevent sagging, which puts an additional strain on the back muscles. In addition, a home pelvic traction set was provided for her to use from time to time.

This treatment was so successful that Olga was back to work about four weeks after her initial attack. She was a typical case of a herniated lumbar disc that responded to conservative treatment. Many cases of low back sprain will respond favorably to heat, muscle relaxant drugs, exercises, and to gentle chiropractic manipulation. Even acupuncture will help to relieve some of the pain in such cases.

An extremely important point in this case is that Olga's cure might well have proven temporary. I say this because of her mental attitude when she left the hospital.

Olga Had to Learn to Relax

After she left the hospital, Olga's biggest problem was fear. She was deathly afraid that she would hurt her back again and have to undergo surgery. Fortunately, her family doctor understood her reaction and was able to allay Olga's morbid fear of a relapse.

His advice to her will also help you:

• He added additional isometric exercises to the ones Olga had learned in the hospital. (The value of exercises will be discussed more fully in a later chapter of this book; they are extremely important. In fact, a newspaper article appearing in November 1973 quoted a former close associate of the late President John F. Kennedy to the effect that exercises helped Kennedy's back condition more than any other single treatment.)

• The doctor explained to Olga that her back, like the rest of her body, reacts to emotional stress and worry. Olga admitted that she had been tense and had slept poorly for weeks before her acute bout of back pain. She was helped to relax by a routine of taking two aspirins in warm milk along with a warm bath before bedtime.

• He urged her to swim more often and to try to reduce the tensions of her job and her life problems.

• Most of all he allayed her damaging fear by assuring her that only a few cases of low back pain require operations. Her chances of needing one were less than one in a thousand.

After this advice was given and taken, Olga learned to live with her occasional backaches.

Some Lessons to Be Learned from Olga's Case

• Perhaps the most important thing Olga learned from her injury is *not to panic.* Her fear as her pain increased added tensions and strains that made her condition worse. Help was on the way. It just took a little time.

• There is no substitute for the family doctor or the general practitioner. He is the starting point in your medical problems. He will eliminate possibilities and arrive at a conclusion as to whether you need a specialist, and if so, what kind.

• Don't search the telephone book's yellow pages for a "pain doctor." There isn't any, since pain may come from so many sources, and even teams of sources. These sources may be bacteria, physical reactions, bones or organs out of place, strains, or even self-induced through the patient's mental attitude. Olga's initial symptoms might just as easily have been caused by a kidney stone or even a disease of the spine, instead of the herniated lumbar disc that was finally diagnosed.

• Another important lesson to draw from Olga's case history is that it is fine to consult your neighbors about cake recipes or the best places to buy cars, but shun their advice on health matters. Your family doctor is still the best expert on your physical ills. Trust him.

Help for Your Own Pain Problems

The example of common backache chosen here does not cover all the many details involved in back troubles. More will be covered in a later chapter devoted to backaches. Olga's case was related here in order to point out the main problem that every chronic pain sufferer faces: *Where do I go for help?*

Summary

A chronic sufferer from backache like John F. Kennedy could surely have gotten the services of the finest physicians in the world. Yet when he was supposedly asked by his close associate Theodore Sorensen to recommend a back specialist, the witty president reportedly replied; "Believe me, Ted, there ain't no back specialists."

In the past ten years a group of specialists have been

emerging who could almost be called pain doctors. Perhaps, in the future, many such physicians will be available. But the chances seem unlikely, for pain is a symptom. There is no disease called pain. Pain is a natural warning to nag us into doing something about a bodily malfunction before it kills us. In this respect, pain is a blessing and a lifesaver. This does not mean that pain must be endured. Once it has served its purpose in warning us and prodding us into taking action, there is no longer any point in suffering. However, since pain can be caused by so many different sources, there will always be a need for the multidisciplinary or team approach to the problem of relieving pain.

You, the patient, are an important member of that team. You can and must help yourself, whether you suffer from headache, neck, arm, or low back pains, painful menstruation, neuralgias and neuritis, arthritis, or from pains associated with cancer. It is much easier to help yourself if you understand something about what pain is, how the nervous system carries the pain signals to the brain, and the psychology of pain as it affects a sufferer. Then we can delve into the specific causes of pain and determine what you and your doctor can do about bringing you new hope for relief from pain.

2

THE ANATOMY
OF PAIN

What is pain?

A little girl, answering this question in her health class examination, gave as good an answer as any dictionary ever did. She said, "It's something that *hurts.*"

It's hard to improve on her answer, but to make things official, let's look it up in *Webster's Dictionary.* The word *pain* is derived from the Latin word *poena* and the Greek word *poine,* meaning *fine* or *penalty.* In modern usage the dictionary says that pain is "an unpleasant or distressing sensation due to bodily injury or disorder." The second meaning is "acute mental or emotional distress or suffering."

You will notice that there are two aspects of pain. One is physical, which produces unpleasant or distressing sensations. The other aspect is in the mind, producing emotional or mental distress.

There are two other words that bear upon our subject. One is *suffering.* The other is *patient.* The word *suffering* means "bearing under." A person who has a constant pain is certainly bearing under it. Doctors refer to their clientele as patients. The word itself, according to Webster, has two meanings. One is "an individual awaiting or under medical care and treatment." The other meaning is "bearing pains or trials calmly and without complaint."

So patients are those who see physicians because they are having to bear under the trials of an unpleasant or distressing sensation due to bodily injury or disorder. There have been people in this situation as long as there have been people. Pain began, according to the Book of Genesis, in the Garden of Eden, where Eve was condemned to "bring forth your children in pain," (Gen. 3:16) because of her sin of disobedience. The desire to alleviate pain goes back to Genesis as well, for it is described that "The Lord God caused a deep sleep to fall upon Adam, and he slept, and he took one of his ribs and closed up the flesh instead, thereof." (Gen. 2:21) This would tend to indicate the first anesthesia.

Today, anyone can pick up a book and study diagrams of the human body that show parts of the brain, spinal cord, and nerves and give simple explanations of how a nerve impulse can travel from a finger to the brain cortex. But primitive man had no way of transmitting knowledge except by word of mouth, for the art of writing was unknown until about 10,000 years ago. Despite the handicap of not being able to record his discoveries, prehistoric man had a tremendous gift of observation and a remarkable imagination. He realized that there was a definite cause behind every action, and his imagination developed explanations for all that he observed.

Today, many of these explanations appear ridiculous, especially those that explain pain in terms of demons, worms, and other strange forces working inside the body. Many of these beliefs survived when man learned how to read and write. In the early books of the Egyptians, descriptions can be found of special demons who cause particular ailments. For example, a toothache was described as being caused by the gnawing of a worm, and jaundice was believed to be caused by a demon that made the body yellow and the tongue black. However, if one substitutes the word *bacteria* for *demons*, the Egyptians were not far wrong.

In more primitive tribes, magic rituals were set up and administered by witch doctors, who were thought to have special powers to drive pain-causing demons from the human body. While this part was pure superstition, the primitive medicine man had a remarkable knowledge of the use of herbs and natural substances to relieve pain and effect cures. He knew about the medicinal uses of opium and mandrake root as painkillers. Quinine, used in treating malaria, was used first by the Indians of South America. And in India and South Africa primitive tribes use infusions of willowbark to relieve joint pains. Chemists have shown that this willowbark contains salicylic acid, a constituent of aspirin. Another classic example of an old folk medicine that has proven its worth in modern medicine is Rauwolfia, an herb used in India since ancient times. It was shown to have remarkable power to control blood pressure, as well as to calm emotional tensions. It has been purified and sold in its pure form as Reserpine.

Egyptian Painkillers

Three thousand years before Christ, the Egyptians developed a remarkable knowledge of anatomy. The *Edwin Smith Surgical Papyrus* (1600 B.C.), an early medical treatise found in a tomb, shows that they also knew methods of relieving pain during operations. It is incredible to read that the Egyptian physicians used pressure on the carotid arteries to produce unconsciousness. These are two large arteries, one on each side of the neck, that carry blood from the aorta—the main artery of the body—to the head and brain. Pressure applied to these arteries reduces the flow of blood to the brain, resulting in unconsciousness. This procedure can be dangerous, especially with older people, since it can result in a stroke or permanent paralysis. For younger patients, however, the technique can be successful, allowing the patient to drop into a temporary unconscious state. This permitted early Egyptian physicians to painlessly open an abscess or amputate a gangrenous limb.

Another significant early medical document is the *Code of Hammurabi* issued in Babylon about 1900 B.C. Actually a code of laws, the wise Babylonian ruler also spelled out the civil responsibility of physicians, their fees, and the specific penalties if they failed to achieve a cure. As an example of a fee, he decreed: "If a physician shall open a cataract with an operating knife and preserve the eye of the patient, he usually should receive ten shekels of silver. . . ."

Chinese Medicine

The Egyptians learned about anatomy from their religious custom of embalming the dead. This involved opening up the body, removing internal organs, and also opening the skull before the corpse was embalmed to make a mummy. They were never terrified at opening corpses as were many ancient people, and as a result, their medicine was based upon solid knowledge of the human body.

The Chinese, on the other hand, contributed much to medicine without an extensive knowledge of anatomy. Confucius, their great sage, considered the human body sacred and taught, in the sixth century B.C., that it should not be violated after death.

Nevertheless, a complicated philosophy of explaining health evolved. Life was explained as *Chi*, governed by the balance and harmony of opposites known as *Yang* and *Yin*. The forces of Yang and Yin flowed throughout the body. Out of this concept, and mainly through trial and error, they developed acupuncture as a technique of inserting needles into various parts of the body to let out excess Yang or Yin.

This achieved a balance between the two "life forces," which make up health.

While we still use many ancient herbs and drugs, acupuncture is the only ancient healing operation that has been revived by modern medicine. By contrast, other methods such as bloodletting, application of leeches, and tonics of sulphur and molasses have long since been discarded.

The Development of Anesthesia

The Greeks and Romans also made contributions to medicine and to the concept of pain, but the greatest single advance in the history of relieving suffering did not come until the nineteenth century, when anesthesia became a reality. Up to this time surgery was a nightmare. The only way a patient could escape the most frightful pain was to faint or get so drunk that he did not know what was going on.

The story of the discovery of anesthesia is a fascinating one itself and has been told many times in colorful ways in books like *Triumph Over Pain* by Rene Fülop-Müller, *Mystery, Magic and Medicine* by Haggerty, and *Victory over Pain* by Victor Robinson.

The discovery of so-called scientific anesthesia was made in a climate of controversy and personal tragedy. Sir Humphrey Davy (1788–1829) of England experimented upon himself by breathing nitrous oxide, the so-called laughing gas. He later reported that the gas "may probably be used with advantage in surgical operations in which no great effusion of blood takes place."

No one tried Sir Humphrey's suggestion, but the gas did become popular as a stimulant. Laughing gas parties were held somewhat in the manner of today's marijuana orgies. In the early part of the nineteenth century, these parties spread from England to the eastern seaboard of the United States. People would inhale the gas to become intoxicated. They would stagger and stumble and otherwise feel good. Many pseudoprofessors of chemistry and side-show itinerants staged these parties. During this period observers noted that people under the influence of laughing gas would stumble against things, hurting their legs, but would not complain of pain.

The breakthrough was made by a dentist named Dr. William Thomas Morton (1819–1868), of Massachusetts, who introduced ether as an anesthetic. Morton had learned about the use of nitrous oxide from a former partner, Horace Wells, a dentist in Hartford, Connecticut, who had used laughing gas in dentistry. One of Wells's patients died, and this caused the dentist to withdraw from practice. Subsequently he ended his life tragically.

The unfortunate experience of his friend, however, did not deter Morton. He was intrigued with the idea of suppressing pain by the use of an anesthetic. He considered laughing gas too dangerous after Wells's experience and began experimenting with ether. Ether is a liquid made by the action of sulphuric acid on alcohol. Its fumes can render a person unconscious.

Later, when Morton was studying medicine, he persuaded the famous Dr. John Collins Warren, the great surgeon of the Massachusetts General Hospital, to allow him to give the new anesthetic a trial in surgical procedures. This famous operation took place in the so-called ether amphitheater of the Massachusetts General Hospital on October 16, 1846. Dr. Warren removed in five minutes a mass from the neck of a patient who felt no pain during the operation. Although this was the first public demonstration of ether as an anesthetic, credit for first using ether in operations belongs to Crawford W. Long, of Georgia, who used it as early as 1842.

Long was reticent about talking of his work, and he also

lacked the great prestige of Dr. Warren. The now famous *New England Journal of Medicine*, then called the *Boston Medical and Surgical Journal*, published an account of the Warren operation in its November 1846 issue. The story of how sulphuric ether had been used to induce anesthesia and eliminate pain electrified the medical profession. This was the birth of modern anesthesia.

Ether rendered the patient unconscious. The next leap forward in the struggle to control pain was the subsequent discovery of local anesthetics. These could be used to reduce pain in small areas. Cocaine was among the first discovered. It was shown by Dr. Carl Koller in 1884 that cocaine, when applied to the eye, blocked pain over the cornea area. This experiment made cocaine practical as an anesthetic for eye operations.

By this time organic chemistry was rapidly advancing. From cocaine, a German chemist, Alfred Einhorn, conceived the idea of synthesizing procaine, known to us today as Novocain. This new anesthetic was easy to inject into various parts of the nervous system, especially the nerve of the face for dental anesthesia, and in 1901, into the spinal canal for surgical operations.

Capsule History of the Discovery of the Nervous System

The development of anesthetics was delayed for centuries because the transmission of nerve impulses throughout the body was not understood. Knowledge of the nervous system was discovered slowly. Our present concepts evolved after electricity was discovered. It then followed that there was a great similarity between the movement of electricity over wires and the movement of impulses through the nerves.

It happened this way: A professor of medicine at the University of Bologna, Luigi Galvani, observed in 1786 that muscles of an animal body would contract when subjected to an electrical current. An interesting story tells how he made this discovery. Galvani, as part of some experiments in his laboratory, had suspended some frogs on copper hooks. Galvani then noticed that when the wind blew the frogs' backs against an iron rail that their legs twitched, even though they were dead. From this Galvani concluded that the contact of the copper hooks and the iron rail produced a current of electricity. He called this phenomenon electricity.

Another Italian, Alessandro Volta, drew the conclusion from Galvani's experience that dissimilar metal, placed in a solution that conducts current, could be made to conduct electricity. This is the basic principle of the storage battery used in automobiles. You will recognize Volta's name in the word *volt*, which is a measurement of electrical pressure.

Hence, between the work of Galvani and Volta, the basic ideas of animal electricity were discovered and elucidated. A half-century later the German physician and physiologist Von Helmholtz succeeded in measuring the speed at which nerve impulses travel. He made other great contributions to electrophysiology. The concept was then firm that an electrical current travels through a nerve to transmit its impulse to the brain.

These basic discoveries that nerves are tissues that conduct electrical impulses revolutionized our concept of the nervous system. Additional discoveries were then made through animal experiments and human observations that nerve impulses travel through the body in different ways to reach the brain. We interpret these impulses as pain.

You may wonder, if we correctly understand the mechanics of pain transmittal, why we cannot control man's pain. This will be possible only when we have a perfect knowledge of the working of the human brain. Then we can possibly think of the brain as a computer that can be programmed to react in different ways to pain.

Just to show you something of the complexity of the problem, imagine at any moment, even while you are reading these words, that you are aware of sitting in a chair, that you have different feelings throughout your body, such as hunger, a desire to urinate, or a desire to get up and walk around. Thus, your brain is carrying on many different lines of thought and activity.

You may also be hearing many sounds, but you block them out as you read and focus your attention on what is written here. This is because man's marvelous brain can control thousands or even millions of impulses that course through the computerlike nervous system every second. And this tremendous amount of work is done in a brain that hardly weighs three pounds.

Pain and Your Nervous System

Now let's take a bird's-eye view of those parts of the brain, spinal cord, and nerves that are used to perceive pain. I shall not go into those parts of your nervous system used to see, hear, taste, walk, or even smell. This simplifies our job because we can focus upon those parts of the nervous system that conduct the nerve impulses that we interpret as pain.

Let's say, for example, that you decide to sit down in a chair. Then you suddenly jump up, screaming, "Ouch! What happened? Who put that blankety-blank tack on my seat?"

Let's examine that behavior. In a split second you have jumped from your chair, yelled out, and dropped your hand to rub the seat of your pants where you felt the pain.

How could all this happen so rapidly? Well, the first impulses were picked up by the skin of your buttock. The impulses passed through the nerves in the skin, traveling by free nerve endings or so-called pain receptors. These free nerve endings are microscopic fibers of nerves that are present in the millions of nerve endings in the skin. The impulses find their way to larger nerves that are visible, and finally they travel through the branches of the sciatic nerves, which are among the largest nerves in the body, into finer nerves in the spinal canal.

This is the path of transmission of the nerve impulse that made you holler "Ouch!" and jump from your chair to rub the seat of your pants. This nerve impulse went from the source of the pain impulse, which in this case was a tack pressing against the skin, to the brain, where it was computer-processed into the sensation of pain. Reaching the brain is only half of the total reaction to the pain of sitting on a tack.

The nerve impulse then reenters the spinal canal and joins the spinal cord segment that controls that part of the body that will react. A relay is then set up and another impulse goes to another nerve that sends a message impulse to your buttock that makes you jump up to remove yourself from the source of your pain.

This is the same *reflex* action that occurs if you place your hand on a hot stove or accidentally put your foot into a tub of hot water.

While this reflex withdrawal of the leg takes place, an impulse is also sent upward to the spinal cord. This is a large cable of nervous tissue protected by the spinal column. The spinal cord connects with the brain at the base of the head. Impulses sent through the spinal cord go into the upper portion of the brain stem, finally ending in a portion of the brain called the thalamus.

The word *thalamus* literally means "seat." It is the main perception center in the brain. From it impulses are routed to various parts of the brain cortex. In the example of sitting on a tack, the impulse may go from the thalamus to the front part of your brain. This makes you aware of the discomfort. At the same time an impulse shoots to the speech center on the left side of your brain (in right-handed people). This causes you to say "Ouch!"

At the same time that your awareness of discomfort makes you jump up, an impulse may go to your emotion center and this causes you to exclaim, "What a stupid jerk I was to sit on a tack!" Or, if you are a worrisome type of person, the impulse registered into the cortex may set up a train of thoughts whereby you may say to yourself, "I wonder if that tack was rusty? Now I may get tetanus."

All of these flashing impulses occurred in a split second. You jumped up automatically without consciously commanding yourself to do so in order to protect yourself because a pain impulse stimulated your brain. At the same time these action impulses were activating your body and speech, impulses also went to the memory portion of your brain to store the painful experience as a lesson for the future.

Just exactly how the brain stores memory and then sets off the memory train when we need it is not completely understood. But we do know that you will not forget immediately the pain of that tack and will be a little careful for some time each time you sit down.

Actually the "wiring of the brain," as a writer once put it, is not yet understood in its entirety. An international symposium of neuroscientists, meeting at the Massachusetts Institute of Technology in 1973, discussed a new concept of brain action. The older concept assigned control of different functions to different and specific portions of the brain. However, it was noted that if portions of the brain were removed, it did not destroy the brain's ability to continue those functions supposedly contained and controlled by the missing portion of the brain.

This change of control was explained by just saying, "Another part of the brain took over the function." However, a new concept discussed at the Massachusetts symposium holds that the various functions are spread all through the brain.

Regardless of which concept is right, the principle remains

the same. Impulses go from the seat of the pain to the brain, where they trigger specific reactions and record a memory trace. Let's review in a simple way the basic nervous structures involved in transmitting a painful impulse.

THE NERVE RECEPTOR

Pain begins with a nerve receptor. You will appreciate that pain is not a precise sensation, such as the precision to know that you have a pain in your hand. It is a diffuse type of sensation. There are actually no special pain receptors as was once thought. Instead there are free nerve endings.

THE PERIPHERAL NERVES

The free nerve endings transmit their impulses to the peripheral (outer or external) nerves. These nerves may be in the skin, but they can also be in our various organs, such as the eye. They can be in ducts inside the body that cause you to have a cramping pain when, for example, a stone lodges in the gall bladder or a terribly colicky pain like that associated with a kidney stone. This pain results from stretching the ureter, the tube that carries urine from the kidney.

From these endings, wherever they may be—in the eye, the skin, or the gut—the impulses are sent to nerves that carry the message to a nerve center. The nerves are large and visible and can be demonstrated by the surgeon or the anatomist. These nerves can measure from a sixteenth of an inch to almost a half-inch in diameter, as in the case of the large sciatic nerve.

From the peripheral nerves themselves, the impulses must

reach the spinal cord and the nerve centers of the brain. They make a connection with a spinal ganglion, which is a nerve center outside the spinal canal, just where the nerve enters the spinal cord. It then goes into the incoming nerve root or the posterior nerve root. This root is the final transmission pathway to the spinal cord.

THE SPINAL CORD

The spinal cord is the main cord of nervous tissue that conducts the impulses from the periphery (by which I mean the skin, gut, or muscles). The impulses in the spinal cord have several pathways to complete their connections. A second nerve relay can then send the impulse outward to the motor nerve to cause a reflex response or withdrawal of an arm or other part of the body, as in the case of touching your finger to a hot stove.

At the same time an impulse crosses over, if you happen to touch your right hand to a hot stove and then withdraw it. The second relay impulses then cross over and go on up the spinal cord into the white matter. The white matter does not have nerve cells but has nerve fibers for transmission of the impulse. The impulses follow these to the end station in the brain.

This pathway of connection through the spine is called the *spinothalamic tract* because it goes from the spinal cord to the thalamus in the brain.

This is just like taking another road to get to a destination. If you were told, for example, that to get to City Hall in your town you should go down Broad Street and make a right turn where it meets Twentieth Street, then go north on Twentieth Street to City Hall, you will have the comparison. By analogy, the connection of Broad Street and Twentieth Street is where the spinal nerve enters and then transmits to the spino-thalamic tract. The thalamus can be thought of as City Hall or our destination.

THE THALAMUS

The thalamus is the end station in the brain for all nerve impulses. This includes not only the impulses that produce the sensation of pain but also those of temperature, hearing, smell, taste, and awareness. The latter would include aware-ness of where your muscles are at any moment and whether they are stretched or relaxed.

From the thalamus, an intricate mass of nerve cells in the center of the brain, impulses are sent to various parts of the brain itself. You might compare the thalamus to a telephone switchboard. It takes incoming calls and routes them to the proper destinations.

THE CEREBRAL HEMISPHERES

Somewhere in the cerebral hemispheres—within the think-ing portion of the brain—are the final ending points of all sensory impulses. Here there is an association, correlation, and interpretation of those impulses that we call pain. Somehow they are all brought together.

Think of the cerebral hemispheres as the Pentagon in Washington, D.C. All the thousands of reports from an end-less number of military outposts come here. Once the mes-sages from the field reach headquarters in the Pentagon, decisions can be made on the basis of these reports. Likewise, when the pain impulses reach the cortex, a decision can be made to holler "Ouch!" or "Damn it!" or "What a fool I was!"

In this chapter we have been concerned with the anatomy and physiology of pain. There is another and equally important side that deals with the psychology of pain. It, too, is essential in understanding what causes pain.

3

THE PSYCHOLOGY
AND MEANING
OF PAIN

The anatomic pathways through which the human being perceives pain are mechanical, forming a living electrical system. As such it should be subject to mechanical laws and to mechanical repair. Repair, however, is complicated, because the human machine is more than a mechanical device. It has emotions ranging from fear to resentment, from happiness to despair. These complicate the purely mechanical functioning of the body.

Psychology, then, becomes an important part of both understanding pain and treating it. Almost every person who suffers from long-standing pain has asked his doctor, "Why do I have to suffer like this?"

The obvious answer, the human body being the machine that it is, would be, "You suffer because something got out of gear in your machine." But this would not be true. Pain, which is a miserable curse to so many chronic sufferers, is also one of mankind's greatest blessings.

The Blessing of Pain

No one who has lived to adulthood can truly say that he has never experienced pain. Most of us, at some point in our lives, have asked ourselves, a doctor, or even Heaven: "Why must I suffer like this?"

The answer is simple enough. Although we complain that our pain is killing us, the basic truth is that if it were not for pain, we would all probably die.

Pain is not a disease in itself. It is not an injury. It is not a malfunction of the body in any way. It is perfectly natural. Pain is a symptom—a sign or natural warning than something is wrong in the human body. In this respect, pain is a blessing and a lifesaver. Without the warning of pain, we could run rusty nails through our feet and walk on whistling until we finally dropped dead of tetanus. An appendicitis attack could go unnoticed until the appendix ruptured and spread poison so thoroughly through the body that nothing could save the patient. A cut could turn into gangrene and cause the loss of a limb. Likewise, the common pains a woman feels in the last days before childbirth are nature's way of warning her to prepare for the delivery of her baby.

If pain is but a signal that something is wrong, it might well be argued by a chronic sufferer that a simple warning is enough. Nerves do not have to nag one to distraction. Unfortunately, the human body was designed for a kind of people and not a single person. While one person might heed a gentle warning, the majority of us must have nagging pains to force us to see a doctor or to do something for ourselves. Pain must be sufficiently severe to force us to heed its warning. Otherwise it fails in its basic purpose.

This does not mean, of course, that agonizing pain must be endured. Once it has served its purpose, it is time to get rid of the agony as quickly as possible.

It is *chronic* pain, then, that is our enemy. This is the kind of pain that comes from incurable ailments and goes on for days and days and weeks and weeks. It is the suffering endured by arthritic patients, cancer victims, and sometimes amputees who have a persisting pain in the stump. And sometimes there is a *phantom pain* in cases like a missing limb. It sometimes amuses people to hear an amputee complain of a pain in his big toe when you both know the big toe isn't there anymore. But it isn't amusing to the victim, and the pain to him is real indeed.

Of course, not all pains are disagreeable. The sensation of hunger is a pain that is not entirely unpleasant when we know that a delicious meal is waiting for us. Without the sensation of hunger we would not enjoy eating. In the same manner, the sensation of thirst is necessary for the enjoyment of drinking. It is when these sensations of hunger and thirst cannot be fulfilled that they become painful and bring on suffering.

The philosophic or religious aspect of pain is an entirely different subject. Pain, as we have seen, is a necessary warning system, but why it is necessary to have the suffering that causes pain is a question that science cannot answer. It is a subject that must be pursued in one's own religious convictions. To go into it here would take us too far afield.

An important point to remember in discussing pain is that we must reckon with the vast differences in pain perception in various individuals. This is true not only in the same race and culture but also in different cultures and races. For example, the Hindus of India often exhibit remarkable ability to suffer pain. We see their religious zealots undergoing what must be frightful punishment as part of their religious vows. The fire-walking ordeals one can see in India, Japan, and the South Seas have considerable trickery connected with them, but when penitents lie on beds of nails, pierce their bodies with sharp instruments, and hang themselves in distorted positions, there is no way for them to escape frightful pain that makes Westerners shudder in horror. In a like manner the Chinese and the American Indian are both famous for their ability to withstand pain without complaining.

The Psychology of Painful Emotions

The nervous pathways through which pain impulses travel are relatively easy to explain compared with trying to discuss the so-called psychology of pain.

The word *psychology* is used in a hundred different meanings. I am using it here to refer to the emotional aspects of pain. Man is made up of a body and an emotional system, or a body, mind, and emotions. This is called a *psychosomatic unit,* meaning a functioning unit. Since emotions are a basic part of a person, we must try to understand that physical pain is not just a matter of an impulse traveling through a nerve into the spinal cord and then into the brain.

Each time we feel pain—for example, a severe toothache—there is the counterpart of an emotional reaction. This is what makes pain so different in the human being, as compared with lower animals. Animals have toothaches too, but they do not suffer with them as much as we do. This is because they only suffer from the pain, while human beings suffer from both the pain and the emotional disturbances that the pain brings with it. Suppose that your dog or cat or other favorite pet has a toothache over the weekend. Can you imagine it complaining to you that the pain spoiled his Fourth of July outing? Can you imagine it expressing its irritation because it could not find a dentist during the holiday?

An animal may howl and whimper, but it is all due to pain. Man's emotions and imagination cause him to build up an emotional response to his pain, such as anger because he can't find a dentist when he needs him or resentment because the toothache prevented him from having a good time at the Fourth of July picnic. It might even be bitterness because he had to be the only one in misery at the gay affair. In any case, his original pain has now been multiplied by his emotional reactions to the original suffering.

It is important to note that there is no particular set of emotions inherently associated with pain. The pain impulses only sound a sharp warning that something is threatening the human body. Once the brain becomes aware of this threat, the emotions react with anger, resentment, impatience, and, in some cases, downright fear. The exact reaction varies with individuals according to their emotional and psychological makeup.

Many times I have had to tell patients with chronic backaches that they would just have to endure their pain while methods were worked out to help them. Many of them have exclaimed: "But, doctor, I can't stand this any longer! I'm afraid to move for fear I'll hurt my back. I can't do *anything*. I can't work. I can't even *live!*"

The key phrase in this statement is, "I'm afraid to move for fear I'll hurt my back." Even though I have explained that there is a new hope for sufferers from chronic pain, when I add that it will take time to find a method of relief the patient all too often reacts with fear. The realization that there is no magical way to relieve his suffering makes him wonder if I have been honest in claiming that there is hope for him. He sees the distinct possibility that he may have to live with his pain indefinitely.

This is a simple and human reaction—an emotional reaction that is followed by anger, resentment, and sometimes depression. We look at those about us who are not suffering and ask ourselves, "Why does it have to be me?"

This question is not asked in a dispassionate way. The speaker is suffering. He cannot pass his hurt on to someone else. Doctors, friends, and loved ones may try to help, but in the end pain is an experience that each of us must bear alone.

How many times have parents, loving husbands, and wives expressed their wishes to take on the pain and suffering of an afflicted loved one? But this can never happen except in legend. One such story concerns Babur the Tiger, a warrior king who founded the Mogul Empire in India. In 1530 A.D. Babur's beloved son Humayun was dying. The ruler consulted all the doctors in his realm without success. Finally a seer told him that the prince would not recover until he gave away the thing he loved most.

"My son loves me most of all things in the world," Babur replied quickly. He then circled the sick prince's bed, crying to heaven to let him take Humayun's sickness into his own body. From that exact instant, the story claims, the prince began to improve and his father began to waste away. Within three months the son was cured and the father was dead. And it is said that Babur died with a smile on his lips.

There is no other record of a loved one taking on the suffering of his beloved. And we may wonder about the truth of this one, although it is an historical fact that Babur did waste away as his son recovered from a serious illness. In the main, however, we can depend upon the doctor's skill, a nurse's ministrations, and our loved one's support and help, but in the dark of the night we must suffer our pain alone. According to Ivan Pavlov, the renowned behaviorist, we are conditioned to react to pain in a certain way. In this regard we can do much to help ourselves to bear our pain when outside help has done all it can. And one of the best ways we can help ourselves is to learn *not to panic.*

It is easier not to panic if we force ourselves to learn that pain is something that can be handled. We must continue to seek out a physician who not only understands our condition but who can get to the seat of our pain. When you can do this, you have come a long way toward eventual relief.

Now let's take a further look at painful emotions. Earlier we mentioned that pain gives rise to emotional reactions that supplement the basic pain and often increases our misery. But it is also common for emotional reactions to come first and cause pain themselves.

Painful emotions do not cause the type of pain we experience with a toothache or a strained back. It is purely mental in its origin. Let us take as an example the sudden death of a dearly beloved. We experience grief, anguish, and sometimes resentment—basically the same emotions we get from our physical pain. These emotions are no less painful because they are mental rather than physical in origin.

The realization that we will never again see a loved one can cause some of us to become so depressed and distraught that we also wish to die. This same suicidal impulse may come from emotional pain from disappointments in love, from severe financial losses, feelings of being unwanted, and from many other things that deeply affect one's emotions. This pain is caused by man's emotional counterpart to his bodily function.

Unnatural Pains

We all know people who strike us as oddballs because they enjoy pains. There are varying degrees of these pain lovers. In a milder form it may be the wife of a neighbor who seems to enjoy being sick and whose greatest pleasure appears to be relating her symptoms to all who will listen. In its most severe form pain-loving people get a special kick in their twisted emotional lives by seeking out pain and suffering. These people are masochists who have sexual aberrations that cause them to get intense pleasure from being whipped.

On the other hand, there are sexual deviates who delight in causing pain to others. These are sadists. They delight in watching others suffer and love to inflict harm to the point of hearing another person scream in agony. The recent motion picture *A Clockwork Orange* showed some of this type of abberation.

Summary

Man experiences pain in a special way because his emotional life is the counterpart of his physical function. His physical pain, whether caused by neuritis, arthritis, or an injury, is accompanied by an emotional reaction that produces a peculiar pain of its own. This emotional reaction causes him to experience shock, bewilderment, fear, anguish, and grief. In addition, chronic pain, because of its enduring nature, also causes its victims to develop depressed resentful attitudes.

Those who triumph over chronic pain have taken advantage of the psychology of emotions. They have conditioned themselves to be sensitive to accept the pain in a special way that causes them to develop a higher threshold for it.

4

HOW DOCTORS FIND THE CAUSES OF YOUR PAIN

1814356

Clinical tests and a recitation of your symptoms are valuable aids to your doctor in determining the cause of your pain. But the story of your life may help him just as much. This is because of the vital part played by the emotions in any kind of severe pain.

For example, let's consider the case of Virginia. Her history from the cradle up was that of a go-getter. Virginia was a hard-driving woman who knew what she wanted and went after it with all the energy at her command. This is fine, up to a point. When I first came to know her, Virginia was a handsome woman in her late thirties with drive and ambition that never permitted her to rest or settle for anything less than the best. She had been this way all her life, never content to run with the pack. She had to be out in front. In high school she had been president of her class and the valedictorian, and during her two years in junior college she excelled in all her subjects.

At this time she made two decisions. One was that she didn't need to "waste more time in school," as she put it, and that Bill, a fellow student, was the man she wanted to share the rest of her life with. She quit school and went to work in a bank. Her intense drive caused her to rise rapidly. Within ten years she had moved from clerk to teller to assistant cashier and finally to vice-president in charge of commercial loans.

This is an important and time-consuming job. Yet along her busy way to the top Virginia managed to give birth to two sons, spaced three years apart, run her household efficiently, and still find time for the Cub Scouts and other civic functions.

Then, after she passed thirty-five, this dynamo of energy started complaining of daily headaches. In the beginning they came on in the morning, striking over her forehead. By the end of the day the pain spread over her entire head. At first she thought the pain was due to a recent hysterectomy she had undergone. The change in her female glands was causing the trouble, according to several doctors whom she consulted. They predicted that the pains would subside once her body adjusted to its new condition. She gulped aspirin without results and waited for the headaches to go away.

When this did not happen, Virginia joined the medical merry-go-round club. She sought advice from everyone and got help from no one. Her friends insisted that her headaches were caused by disgust with having to work. One neighbor insisted that this had to be the basis, because she had an aunt whose friend had the same condition. Another confided in a conspiratorial whisper that the real trouble was her suppressed dislike of her husband. "I know," her informant said. "I have the same trouble." None of these and similar "diagnoses" impressed Virginia. She thoroughly enjoyed her work and loved her husband and family.

Giving up on getting medical advice from friends, Virginia also got no relief from her family doctor. He treated her with medications and made studies to check for low thyroid secretions.

Worried now that there might be pressure on her brain, the doctor sent Virginia to a medical neurologist. He made a series of tests involving reaction of the pupils of her eyes and the muscles of her face. They checked out within normal limits. The movement in her arms and legs was examined. Her reflexes were shown to be present and equal. This indicated that her brain and nervous systems were working satisfactorily.

When the doctor told her so, Virginia replied irritably, "If everything is so perfect, why do I have these terrible headaches all the time?"

"In this kind of trouble," he said, speaking carefully, "it is easier to determine what isn't causing the pain than it is to determine what is. But by eliminating those things that are not the cause, we'll eventually narrow down the source of the trouble.

"I am certain that you don't have to worry about a possible brain tumor," he went on. "My neurologic examination indicates that everything is working all right. This diagnosis is supported by your skull X rays, which show nothing wrong. And as a final check, you had a special brain scan test that makes use of atomic particles. It verifies the other examinations. You do not have a tumor or anything seriously wrong in your brain."

Virginia sat stiffly in her chair, staring impatiently at the doctor as he spoke. Her hands kept clicking and unclicking the catch on her handbag. When he finished speaking, she said, "Well, what *have* I got! And more importantly, what can I do about it?"

Thinking over her negative tests and taking note of her history while observing her tenseness, he said, "Most likely your headaches are caused by severe emotional tension."

She exploded, jumping angrily to her feet. "That is absolutely ridiculous!" she snapped. "Others have tried to tell me the same stupid thing. I am not troubled by nerves and I never have been."

She flounced out of the office and did not come back. In her continuing search for help, she consulted a local chiropractor. His manipulations brought her some relief, but not enough. The pains continued. Then, when acupuncture became news, Virginia eagerly sought this exotic new treatment. It helped some, but again the relief was insufficient. At this state she finally gave up, convinced that nothing could help her. It appeared that she was doomed to live with her throbbing head for the rest of her life.

What We Can Learn from Virginia's Case

Virginia went through the legitimate routines of medical doctors but found no magical relief. Sometimes, as doctors, we have to admit that we cannot remove all types of pain. We hope, however, to control it sufficiently that we can offer enough relief to the patient that life becomes bearable.

In Virginia's case her condition was complicated by her refusal to face the truth. This was simply that she could not continue to drive herself at thirty-five the way she could at eighteen. The number is legion who have told their doctors, "But it can't be *that*. I've done that all my life, and it never hurt me." There comes a day in all of our lives when we can no longer do all the things we did in former years. It is tragic how so many refuse to face up to this reality.

It was only after Virginia was finally able to bring herself to this realization that she found relief from her pain. Her trouble, as several doctors had tried to tell her, was chronic tension that tightened her neck muscles, causing pressure that generated her throbbing migraine headaches.

Her eventual treatment began with a series of physical therapy routines to relax the muscles in the back of her neck. This also included some injections into the muscles to help them relax after so many years of constant tenseness. After that her treatments were more self-help than anything else. She received guidance and help from her doctor, but the basic element in her improvement came as she learned to take things more easily and to avoid the buildup of everyday tension. She had to stop racing through life.

How Doctors Study a Pain Problem

Virginia's tenseness was clearly apparent to every doctor she visited. However, it would have been a serious mistake for them to have diagnosed her condition on this alone. Anyone is going to be tense and irritable if they are in pain. First, exhaustive tests had to be made to rule out all possibility of more serious trouble. Once this was done, her history of long years of tension-producing activity became an important clue.

History-taking then is a basic essential of getting to the bottom of chronic pain problems. The questions that doctors ask often seem bizarre to their patients. This is especially true when the questions involve something that occurred back in one's childhood. You may wonder what difference it makes if you had scarlet fever as a child when you are seeking aid for an adult heart condition. When your doctor asks such questions, he is probing the past for something that might be the seed of your current problem. Having rheumatic fever as a child has a tendency to harm the heart valves. Later, rheumatic fever can become the basis for adult heart trouble. In the same manner, a person exposed to poliomyelitis before the Salk vaccine could develop a limp later in life because of a weak leg.

History-taking is also most important in helping us understand any predisposition to certain types of pain. Migraine headaches, for example, do occur in families. The same is true of high blood pressure. Diabetes also may have a tendency to be passed along to succeeding generations. So both the patient's past history and his family history are clues to the doctor.

History-taking is followed by a general body or physical examination. In addition to the standard thumping, listening to the heartbeat, and making you say "Ahhh," your doctor can tell a lot about your condition just from looking at you. The way you walk, talk, hold yourself, and handle your extremities all are clues to whether your suffering is severe, moderate, mild, or chronic. If you come into the office bent over, this can be a clue that trouble in the spine is compressing a nerve root or causing a spasm in a muscle. Limitations of finger, wrist, elbow, or shoulder movements can be telltale signs of arthritis or muscle irritation. Deep lines under the patient's eyes may indicate a chronic condition. Of course, these and other outward appearances are suggestions to your doctor, rather than positive signs of any particular condition.

The Neurological Examination

Since pain perception is so deeply involved in the nervous system, a neurological examination is a vital part of a study, if your problem is chronic pain. The central nervous system cannot be seen. It cannot be felt. There are peripheral nerves that can be touched under the skin. The nerve behind the elbow is an example. This is the ulnar nerve. When your elbow is banged, the ulnar nerve sends a tingling feeling into your arm and elbow. This is why it is popularly known as the funny bone.

The brain itself cannot be seen. Neurologic specialists must learn about it and other functions of the nervous system through specialized tests. Let's say you have a neurological examination because of a chronic headache or a pain in the face along the lower jaw.

The examination actually begins when you walk into the specialist's office. He will observe how you walk, whether your stride is brisk or dragging, and the movements of your body. Then, by talking to you, he quickly learns if you are fully conscious of your surroundings or whether you are confused. A few direct questions can tell him immediately whether you are aware of time and place. Memory can be tested superficially by asking a few questions about current events. These questions establish the condition of your mind and your perception.

When this general condition examination is complete, the next step is to test the cranial nerves. The head, or cranium, has twelve major nerves. Several of these serve special senses, including vision, hearing, smell, and taste. We can tell a lot about the functioning of these nerves by checking the senses that they serve. For example, if we flash a bright light into the eye, the pupil of the eye will constrict; that is, the iris will close up. Or it may fail to close if something is wrong in the nerve. Thus, the action of the pupil tells a great deal about the functioning of the third cranial nerve and the second cranial nerve as well. Likewise, the movement of the eyes indicate that several of the twelve cranial nerves are working.

The ophthalmoscopic examination comes next. This is a unique and fascinating examination because it permits your doctor to look into the back of your eye for evidence of disorders that would appear to be far removed from your vision. He uses a bright lighted instrument call an ophthalmoscope, which permits him to view the blood vessels that come out of the retina of your eye. The retina is the inner membrane at the back part of the eyeball and contains a layer of cells sensitive to light. These cells change light into nerve impulses, which the optic nerve then carries to the brain, permitting us to see.

In addition to seeing the blood vessels in the retina, the ophthalmoscope shows the optic nerve itself. This is the only place in the entire body where a living part of a nerve can be seen. If the edges of this nerve of vision are blurred, it may indicate pressure inside the head, which could account for headaches. If the blood vessels show nicking or hemorrhages, it may indicate high blood pressure or the effects of diabetes. Thus, the neurologist can tell a great deal about the functioning of the brain from inspecting the eye.

Other cranial nerves can be tested by having the patient close his eyes tightly and stick out his tongue. Feeling in the face is tested with a piece of cotton and also with a pin. Hearing is easily checked with a tuning fork or the tick of a watch.

The motor system of the body is evaluated by asking the patient to open and close his fists and to extend his arms. By asking him to take a few steps back and forth, the doctor can note the gait, which tells a great deal about muscle power as well as coordination.

Finally, the body's reflexes are examined with the use of a little rubber hammer. This is the part often used in movies and on TV. It always makes the audience laugh when the specialist taps his patient's knee with the rubber hammer and the leg kicks out. This is called a reflex, because it cannot be controlled under normal circumstances.

What Does Neurologic Testing Tell the Doctor?

All of these tests are performed to see how the nervous system works. Much of it is indirect examination—something like a mechanic giving a car a road test. He checks it out not by tearing into it but by using his experience to observe how it is running. So, too, a neurologic specialist can tell if your nervous system is functioning properly by observing the results of these tests.

The Value of Special Tests

X-RAY EXAMINATION

Since the ability of a doctor to see disease is extremely limited, we are fortunate to have recourse to X rays for examining the interior of various parts of the body. Unfortunately, X rays have been overrated in their capacity to reveal all types of disease. Many patients with abdominal or chest pains have had complete X rays made of their entire bodies, without ever finding the cause of their discomfort.

Nevertheless, the X-ray examination is of vital importance and should never be omitted. Sometimes the results are negative. At other times they may pinpoint the trouble clearly. Occasionally, they will reveal a totally different source of trouble. I recall one case where a patient complained of chronic chest pains. He was scared to death about having heart trouble. Chest X rays disclosed nothing to cause his pain, but a complete body X ray showed some arthritic changes in his spine. It was pain from this condition that he had misinterpreted as chest pains. They actually came from the back rather than the chest itself.

ATOMIC PARTICLE TESTS

This is what is called radioisotope testing. As a result of nuclear studies following development of the atomic bomb in World War II, scientists became aware that atomic particles could be used to test various functions of the body. These particular particles are called isotopes and are atomic elements with a slightly different mass from the normal element. They can be used for tracing their movement through the human body, because they give off minute amounts of radiant energy that can be measured.

Let me give an example of a practical use of these radioisotopes to study the thyroid gland. This large ductless gland lies near the Adam's apple and controls growth in the body. It can be felt when you swallow. To do this, place your fingers over your Adam's apple and swallow. You can barely feel the thyroid gland.

If your doctor suspects thyroid gland trouble, he will place radioisotopes of iodine in a liquid and give this to you to drink. The atomic particles will be absorbed into your blood through your normal digestive process. While in your body, the radioisotopes will continue to give off their minute quantities of radiant energy. These can be measured with a Geiger counter. Radioactive materials give off radiant energy in same way that a hot stove radiates heat. This radiant energy causes a clicking sound in the Geiger counter. Thus, by holding the pickup unit of the counter against the outside of the body, we can follow the course of the iodine isotopes through the bloodstream. They will travel through the body and enter the thyroid gland, because the thyroid gland picks up iodine. In fact, it is an iodine deficiency in the body that causes an enlargement of the thyroid known as goiter.

By tracing the path of the iodine particles through the thyroid, we can build up a picture of the inside of the gland. It is easy then to determine if there is a small growth or tumor developing in the thyroid. We can also tell from the sluggish movement (or no movement at all) whether the thyroid is working sufficiently. It may not be putting enough of its secretions into the blood, which may be why you feel tired all the time. You can also feel tired because the gland is overworking. In this case the body is somewhat like the engine of your car. You are racing your engine, and that, too, may be why you are so fatigued. All this can be seen in the radioisotope tests, worked out from the clicks of the Geiger counter as the special particles of iodine weave their way through the gland.

This radioisotopic test is also valuable in studying the brain. In this respect it is probably the most useful single test that has become available to us in the last fifteen years. The radioisotope brain scan can give us valuable information that will eliminate the possibility of a tumor of the brain, or of a blood clot on the brain.

The dangers of radioactivity have been stressed so strongly in popular writings that patients often become alarmed when told that radioactive materials are going to be introduced into their bloodstreams. There is no danger whatsoever in the use of radioisotopes. The test is absolutely safe and harmless and is now a part of the routine study of all patients who complain of chronic headaches. While these tests may not determine the cause of your suffering, they permit the doctor to eliminate possibilities. And, if the headache pain is caused by a brain tumor or clot, then it permits treatment early with greatly increased chances of recovery.

SPECIAL X-RAY TESTS

Ordinary X rays are not true photographs. The rays pass entirely through the subject and are recorded on photographic film as a shadowgram. Some parts of the body are harder for the rays to get through than others, and it is this difference that makes up the final X-ray film. In many cases the X rays pass through different organs with the same ease. In these cases the differences in the organs do not show on the X-ray films.

This limitation cuts down the effectiveness of X rays as a means of diagnosing some troubles. We run into this limitation if we use an ordinary X ray, for example, to study your spine in the case of a low back pain complaint. There would not be sufficient contrast between the parts of the body to show if a disc had slipped out of place between the vertebrae and was causing pain by pressing on nerves in the spinal cord.

Fortunately, there is a standard technique we can use to overcome this limitation. This is a special type of X-ray test called the myelogram. It is especially valuable to a specialist who is trying to find out why you have a chronic pain in the back that is also radiating pain into your leg or sciatica.

This is the way a myelogram is taken: A needle is placed into the spinal canal by lumbar puncture in your lower back. The skin, of course, is first anesthetized or "frozen" by a local anesthetic, much like a dentist freezes your gum before he drills your teeth. The needle is a special hollow one, and when inserted into the spinal canal by an expert, there is just a mild discomfort. The needle is used to withdraw fluid from the spinal canal and then used to insert two teaspoons of an oily iodine compound called Pantopaque into the fluid space of the spinal canal.

The Pantopaque material casts a shadow on the X-ray film, giving a beautiful view of the spinal canal. This will show a ruptured disc or compression caused by a spinal cord tumor, either of which could be the cause of the spinal and sciatic pain in the lower back and in the leg.

I recall a patient named Harry who complained of severe pain under his left breast. Harry, who was fifty-four, was sure that he was having a heart attack. A succession of doctors examined his heart and assured him that it was functioning very well for a man of his age. Harry, with the evidence of his chronic pain to support him, refused to accept their diagnoses. He was convinced that he had severe angina and would soon die, because nobody would believe him and do anything for him.

One of his doctors, believing that there might be a neurological basis for Harry's troubles, sent him to me. The neurologic examination that I gave showed that Harry had a loss of feeling over the skin under his left breast. Something some-where was blocking the feeling impulses picked up by the nerve ends in the skin so that they were not reaching the thalamus in the brain. The loss of feeling, I found, extended from the middle of his back around the left side of his chest to the middle of the chest.

This, plus some reflex changes, made me suspect that Harry might have a small tumor pressing the nerve that exits from the spinal canal in the fifth, sixth, and seventh thoracic (between the neck and the abdomen) area.

He was given a myelogram test. It showed a definite defect in this area, indication that there was some compression there. I performed a laminectomy (an operation to remove the bony roof of the spinal canal) and found a benign tumor the size of a soft cherry. This was easily removed and Harry's pain was totally relieved.

Without the myelogram test it would have been impossible to have pinpointed Harry's trouble so easily. Even if a doctor suspects the presence of a tumor, as I did with Harry, the pain is spread over such a wide area that it is difficult without a myelogram test to know the exact location of the trouble. This is why you sometimes hear of "exploratory operations." This means that the exact source of the trouble cannot be found and one or more operations are necessary to find the source. It is quite possible that without the myelogram test Harry could have become totally paralyzed before the cause of his pain could have been discovered.

The situation is somewhat like that of an ulcer patient. Today, barium swallows are used to study the stomach in the same manner as Pantopaque was used in Harry's spinal canal. Before these special X-ray techniques were developed, precise diagnosis would have had to wait until the patient had a ruptured ulcer and almost died. In fact, many did—perhaps as many as 15 percent. So you can see how much this scientific development has done to bring new hope to people suffering from chronic pain.

ELECTRONIC TESTS

In 1924 Dr. Hans Berger invented the electroencephalograph. This mouth-filling name simply means that Dr. Berger's device measures electrical waves given off by the brain. These brain waves are so small that they could not be measured until the invention of the amplifier tube used in radio and television.

In principle, the electroencephalograph is a lot like the electrocardiograph, which is used to check the human heart. Wires are put over the scalp to collect the minute waves, which are then amplified and recorded so the doctor can compare their patterns with those of normal brain waves. The electroencephalograph is helpful with cases of chronic headache to rule out suspicion of pressure on the brain or even a form of epilepsy that could be causing the never-ending pain and suffering.

The test is safe. The only inconvenience is the wires that are placed in the scalp either with fine pins or with a paste material. The test generally requires from about forty-five minutes to an hour to complete.

NERVE BLOCKS TO STUDY PAIN

Let's say that you have severe pain in the cheek. It is in that portion of your face under the eye and extends into the upper lip on the right side. The pain is short lasting but has become so severe that you feel you cannot tolerate it.

You see a pain specialist during one of these attacks. He tells you that the pain is a facial neuralgia. You ask what neuralgia is and are told that it is pain within a nerve or nerves. In other types of pain the nerves merely carry the impulses to the brain to tell of pain somewhere in the body. In neuralgia, the pain originates inside the nerve itself.

Facial neuralgia is a diagnosis that cannot be made by any of the special tests that I have described before. But there is a way to determine if this pain is a true neuralgia that will respond to specific drugs. This is the nerve block test that is made by injecting a small amount of Novocain into the nerve of the cheek. This can be done by a specialist in anesthesia or by a neurologic specialist or even a dentist.

The Novocain will temporarily numb the area around its injection. If the pain disappears during the time the local anesthetic is effective, this is indirect proof that the pain is a neuralgia, rather than caused by a tumor or something else outside the numbed area.

The nerve block test can be used in many parts of the body. Suppose you have severe pain over the left side of your chest and your doctor, like Harry's, is convinced that you do not have heart trouble. Sometimes a series of nerve blocks in the back—where the nerves exit from the spine—will determine whether you have neuritis of the nerves under the ribs.

Many times injections of Novocain into a painful muscle will relieve pain also.

Psychological Aspects of Pain and How to Study Them

In talking about the psychology of pain a little earlier, I mentioned that pain thresholds differ in different individuals. Some people can stand large amounts of pain, while others can barely tolerate the slightest amount of it. This is also true of noise. You may be married to someone who can fall asleep in a crowded room with the radio blaring away, while poor you cannot sleep if you hear the ticking of a watch.

This varying tolerance to pain can take some peculiar deviations, and the psychological aspects of pain have to be taken into account. It is often useful to have a patient undergo a battery of psychologic tests called MMPI (Minnesota Multiphasic Personality Inventory). This is a series of questions designed by experts so that the answers indicate the personality type of the patient.

Suppose you are suffering from a chronic pain in the right side of your abdomen, much like Mildred. According to her early medical history, Mildred became convinced that she had appendicitis. Several doctors assured her that her appendix was quite normal. She refused to believe them. Some time passed and Mildred had an operation to remove her appendix. For two weeks after her recovery Mildred went around telling friends how great she felt and how crazy her doctors had been to try and tell her that her appendix was normal. She declared that she was entirely free of pain for the first time in years.

But a few weeks later Mildred was suffering again. This time she was sure that her ovaries were at fault. Once again she ignored her doctor's advice and had one of her ovaries removed. It did have a tiny cyst on it, but this was not sufficient to explain her piercing pain.

Again she felt great for a short time. Then her old pain returned. She had a hysterectomy and followed this with a series of abdominal operations. Not a single one brought her more than a few weeks' relief. Mildred then decided that her numerous operations had scarred her bowels, making her susceptible to bowel blockage. She became frightened each time she felt a little nauseated and would rush to the hospital, sometimes at two or three in the morning, for reassurance that her bowels were not blocked.

Finally Mildred got a doctor who insisted that she undergo a complete psychological evaluation. The Minnesota Multiphasic Inventory showed that she had a personality that demanded she suffer. The only time that she felt loved and wanted was when she was receiving medical attention.

A recitation of this kind of case shocks people. They think them incredible, but I can assure you that they are not uncommon. Peculiar indeed are the things that disturbed personalities will do or attempt to do. In Mildred's case, she was not consciously faking her suffering. She felt her pain, and she was sincere in her mistaken beliefs as to the origin of her misery.

The question comes naturally to the mind of any layman hearing of a case like this as to why surgeons went ahead with operations when there was nothing wrong with Mildred except her distorted personality. It is doubtful that they were at fault. History-taking, as I pointed out in the beginning, is the basic tool for helping a patient. Many pains and symptoms cannot be seen or felt by a doctor. He must rely on what his patient tells him and modify this by his experience, observations, and clinical tests.

The influence the mind can have over the body is literally amazing. A patient who is absolutely convinced that he or she has a certain disease can often convince his or her body of the same thing, and we see some of the symptoms of that trouble even though the ailment is not there. Perhaps the most common example of this is what we call false pregnancy. Some women, desperately wanting children, actually exhibit some of the symptoms of pregnancy.

Patients like Mildred are certainly in the minority. But because they do exist and since years of struggling with chronic pain can make psychologic changes in the most normal of us, I believe that all patients with chronic pain problems should have careful psychologic evaluations as part of their treatment and diagnoses.

Summary

The search for the causes of your pain include these basic steps:

- *History-taking*, to include not only the case history of

this particular pain but also your childhood medical history and any pertinent major medical problems of your parents;

• *Physical examinations*, to include a careful observation of the way you walk and talk, which can give clues to internal disturbances;

• *Special X-ray tests*, to seek hidden disorders not found by normal X rays and other types of examinations;

• *Psychologic examinations*, to seek clues in the patient's personality which may have a bearing upon his chronic disorders, or detect personality changes that may be coming on because of the constant pain the victim suffers.

5

WHAT YOU
AND YOUR DOCTOR
CAN DO
TO RELIEVE PAIN

So you finally decided to see your doctor. You've put up with your chronic backache or headache too long. By this time you have made the rounds of all the various practitioners, including massage parlors, and you have gotten no help. You have exhausted all the advice of your friends, the drugstore clerk, and ladies and gentlemen on the television commercials. So now that you've at last come to see a doctor, you don't want any more advice, lectures, and stories about people who had "just what you have." You are looking for some real help.

Unfortunately, this is the point where you have to be most careful not to expect miracles. As I pointed out earlier, it takes time to dig out the causes of deep-seated and long-established pain. The best that you can hope for immediately is that your physician will offer you some relief from suffering while he is getting to the bottom of your trouble.

An example is the case of Susan, a perfectly normal, well adjusted person. There was nothing psychotic about her. When she was sick, she was sick. And no nonsense about it. Her trouble started in the shower. She slipped on a piece of soap. In doing so, she twisted her neck and managed to pull some muscles in her neck. The result was severe pain that would not go away.

53

As time passed, she ran the gamut of doctors, receiving a variety of treatments. She was given physical therapy. She received gentle traction on her neck. And she was given a soft cervical (neck) collar that she wore faithfully.

All of these are standard treatments for her type of trouble—but they did her no good. Nor did she get help from the chiropractic manipulations that she took after becoming disillusioned with her other treatments. Her pain increased, leaving her miserable day and night. She began taking extra cocktails at bedtime in an attempt to get some rest. She kept trying to deaden her pain with the bottle until she became a borderline alcoholic.

At last she came under the care of a physician interested in pain control. He put her through the standard examinations. Her reflexes and sensations over her arms and legs indicated that nothing was pressing on her cervical nerve root. Having eliminated this possible source of trouble, her doctor continued probing until he discovered that her fall in the shower had torn a muscle deep in her neck.

This injury should have responded to the conservative treatment she had received from previous doctors but had not done so. Her new doctor found it through a trigger point, which is a highly painful area to the left of her lower neck. He then made some deep injections of Novocain into the area to get down to the injured muscle. The nerve-blocking effects of this local anesthetic brought immediate relief while the drug's effect lasted. The severe pain entirely disappeared after several more injections.

Susan was lucky to obtain relief so quickly. A doctor usually has to spend many hours in preliminary examinations and go through a whole series of treatments before bringing relief to his patient.

Susan's good fortune was that she found a specialist who understood her problem. Such a person is not always easy to find. If your family doctor, your best source of information and help at this initial period, is unable within his experience range to determine the cause of your trouble, then he knows a specialist to whom he can send you.

Then again, symptoms are often so similar for different causes that it is difficult even for an expert to determine quickly if a disorder falls within his specialty or not.

How to Help Yourself During a Pain Crisis

The first thing to bear in mind is that today pain can be relieved. The question of time, however, is a real one. How long will it take? Time seems to magnify when we suffer. Minutes become hours, and hours become days in our minds. This is partly because human beings have imagination and memory. We can recall our past agony and have a tendency to look ahead and panic when we are suffering. You can't wish away or think away a genuine pain. But you can possibly avoid making yourself feel worse than you really need to feel by controlling your imagination.

You can genuinely help yourself if you remember that pain can be relieved in some way. You must retain hope and not lapse into despair. Relief is simply a matter of finding the correct specialist to do it. You must also remember that he may not be able to cure you entirely. You may have to accept a certain amount of pain throughout life, but you can hope to receive from him sufficient easing of your pain to make life liveable.

You may not realize it, but by the new specialist taking a fresh look at your discomforts, you are already assured that something is being done. His thoroughness and review of your complaints in a sympathetic way with a positive attitude should go a long way in making you feel that you will be helped. This renewed confidence in yourself is a genuine help to both you and your doctor.

Drugs and Pain

What part do drugs play in treatment of pain? Many chronic sufferers are convinced that they are of little use. You may have given yourself most of the known drugs on the commercial market or other physicians may have provided them for you. So when your new specialist in pain tells you that you need new drugs, you are sceptical and approach them with a negative attitude. You may have good reason for your lack of faith in drugs, but they do have a place in the control of pain.

One reason for your previous poor results with drugs may have been because they were given to you for what we call symptomatic relief when the cause of the pain could not be discovered. Treating symptoms is like putting salve on small-pox eruptions. It does not get to the core of your trouble. You may have pumped up a low tire, but the nail that causes the leak has not been discovered.

Of course, there are times when treating symptoms is all we can do. You may be one of those patients who does not have something we can isolate and treat specifically. For example, a pain under your right nipple may prove not to be due to a nerve root irritation or a neuralgia that can be cured by an injection in the nerve. Naturally, with the cause of the trouble unknown, any drug used to treat it would be a hit-or-miss situation. So having seen drugs fail in the past, you would naturally be skeptical of the value of any new ones you might be offered.

The unfortunate truth is that there is no single drug known that will offer sufficient relief of pain without causing some unpleasant side effects. I am not speaking about the occasional simple pain in the back, neck, or a headache. We all get these from time to time. One or two aspirins can relieve this discomfort for most people. If you happen to be one of those who are sensitive to aspirin, there are now substitutes you can use that do not irritate the stomach.

If your pain does not respond to the aspirin treatment, stronger medication will be required. Unless the pain can be relieved in a short time by the use of stronger drugs, doctors begin to worry, for you may become accustomed or addicted to the use of drugs.

The drugs used for control of pain so severe it cannot be helped by aspirin include codeine, which is a narcotic and has a side effect, like all narcotics, of producing nausea and constipation. Drugs stronger than codeine include Percodan, Demerol, morphine, and Dilaudid.

Sometimes a drug has to be given by injection because nausea accompanying the pain may be so intense that a patient cannot tolerate the drug in his stomach. There is a false public impression that a drug given by injection will be more effective. This is not so. A drug is given by injection when nausea prevents its use by mouth, and also when drug action is required more rapidly. However, the difference in effective speed between a drug given by mouth and by injection is not as great as it may seem.

Some drugs cannot be given by mouth. Morphine, except in a tincture form where small amounts can be given, is one of these. But Demerol can be given orally with good results.

In addition to pain-killing drugs to relieve or stop pain, doctors like to use combinations consisting of tranquilizing medication or sedatives. These latter drugs calm the anxious patient. Tranquilizers themselves do not control pain, however. Drugs like Miltown, Valium, Phenobarbital, Thorazine, Compazine, and many others known to nonmedical people will not help control pain. Their value is in reducing anxiety with its accompanying tensions and strains, which may have the effect of accentuating the basic pain.

Pessimism about the Control of Pain by Drugs

Any doctor who has worked in the field of pain control sooner or later becomes pessimistic about the use of drugs for pain relief over long periods of time. Drugs can be useful in the beginning of an illness. Indeed, morphine is a blessing if you are suffering severe colicky pains from something like kidney stones. Or, if you have a broken leg and are awaiting treatment, then an injection of morphine is a godsend. However, if such drugs are taken daily, the patient becomes more and more accustomed to their need. The dosage has to be increased. There is nothing more pitiful than seeing a patient who must depend upon morphine and other narcotic drugs for relief of pain on a daily basis.

It is different if a patient has just a month or two to live, because of cancer. Then drugs can be given with increasing dosage without concern. But the solution must be something other than drugs for those who must live out many years with chronic pain.

Physical Treatments for Pain

For centuries civilized man has resorted to some form of physical treatment in addition to drug treatments. Even in the descriptions of ancient Egyptian medicine and other early civilizations we read of hot and cold baths being used for relief of pain and medical treatment. Hydrotherapy, the use of water to soothe painful parts of the body, has been in use for centuries.

Another physical treatment that has only lately come to be appreciated is the ancient form of treatment known as massage. Anyone who has hurt himself or has a pain in his head or neck finds that rubbing the area gives some comfort.

In addition to hot and cold water and massage there are other techniques that use physical measures to fight pain. One of these is electricity in various forms. The passage of a gentle current of electricity through the muscles has been helpful and used since electricity was discovered. Today we have a more sophisticated form of a physical technique in *ultrasound* in which high frequency sound waves are used to break up painful spasms that sometimes occur in the neck and shoulder muscles. Infrared heat lamps that put heat deep into the body muscles also seem to help. The same is true of various traction devices that stretch the neck muscles when we have a sprain in the neck or low back muscles. All of these physical measures have proven helpful in some degree.

Nerve-Blocking Techniques

What happens when a severe pain does not respond to initial treatment with drugs and physical measures? When this happens the specialist in pain control resorts to treatment such as that given to Susan, the woman who hurt her neck after slipping on a piece of soap. You will recall that her treatment involved injections of Novocain into her injured neck muscles.

It is a well-known fact that painful muscles can sometimes be relieved by injections into the nerve that supplies these muscles, if not directly into the muscles themselves. Because of the importance of this treatment, it might be well to discuss it more fully than I did in talking about Susan's case.

Novocain became available for blocking nerves after its discovery near the end of the nineteenth century. Almost everyone has had some experience with it, particularly in dental work. While your jaw was numbed by this local anesthetic, you just felt pressure on your teeth without any painful twinges. The deadened area where the Novocain was effective had a dull or leadened feeling over the lip. Some patients do not like it, but most of us prefer this to the sharp pain of the dentist's drill digging into a throbbing, decayed tooth that is not deadened by Novocain.

Injections of Novocain into painful muscles or into the nerve itself requires skill, and this treatment may be done by a neurologic specialist, an orthopedic surgeon, or an anesthesiologist. There are also many practitioners or family doctors who are skillful in these injection techniques.

One of the most dramatically helpful instances of Novocain injection is in cases involving neuralgia of the face. I recall one elderly patient who came to me with spasms of pain above the right eyebrow. The spasms were so bad that they were driving him crazy. His condition was diagnosed as a supraorbital neuralgia. I will talk about this condition more in a later chapter devoted to neuralgic pains, but I would like here to mention that an injection of a few drops of Novocain into the nerve rapidly released his pain, bringing the patient much relief. When the pain recurred, it was a simple matter to repeat the nerve block by injection. Subsequently, the nerve was destroyed with a few drops of alcohol.

Nerve Surgery for Relief of Pain

Let us say that all these previous techniques—drugs, physical measures, and nerve blocks—have failed to provide permanent relief from your pain. The next step would be to consider cutting the nerve. At this stage of your search for relief from pain you would see a neurosurgeon. Most of the time this type of surgery can be done with predictably good results. However, we are now learning that cutting of nerves is not the final answer for relief of pain, except in clear-cut cases of neuralgia.

You may have heard of people who had achieved dramatic relief of severe sciatic pain after undergoing neurosurgery. This sciatic pain was due to a slipped disc in the spine that failed to respond to physical measures. In such cases, surgical exposure of the nerve root in the lower back and removal of the pressure on the nerve by the slipped or ruptured disc can bring a complete cure. This type of surgery for relief of sciatica can be done with safety.

Surgical relief of pain also has great merit if the patient is suffering from a condition that cannot be cured. Cancer is an example. Let's face it, cancer is a major disease. When it strikes, despite early diagnosis and treatment with cobalt and newer drugs, the malignancy may have spread deep enough to irritate nerve roots and cause constant pain.

An example of what surgery can do to relieve pain in a cancer case is illustrated in the experience of Bill, who developed cancer of the lungs at the age of fifty-five. Bill had been a chronic smoker all his life and irritably rejected all warnings that cigarette smoke was injurious to his health. Shortly after an examination showed that he had cancer of the lung, Bill began to complain of increasingly severe pain in his right hip and leg.

Cancer, unfortunately, is not generally painful in its early stages, frequently permitting a malignancy to spread throughout the body before it is detected. Hence, chances of recovery are greatly reduced. In Bill's case, his neurologic examination suggested that he had pressure on the nerve root. Then, X rays revealed destruction of the bones of his right pelvis, indicating that his cancerous condition had spread into his pelvic bone.

It was perfectly clear at this stage that there was no chance of Bill's recovery. A cancer specialist estimated that he had from four to six months left to live. However, Bill was in excruciating pain from the cancerous growth pressing on nerves in his pelvic region. Even though it would do nothing toward treating his cancer, the doctor suggested that Bill have a percutaneous cordotomy. He explained to his patient that this was the technical name for an operation that consists of passing a fine electrical wire into the spinal cord to knock out the nerves that carry the pain impulses.

He was also careful to explain that this operation would have no effect whatsoever upon the cancer. The surgeon said, "But it will relieve some of your pain and make life liveable again. At one time an operation like this would have taken many hours. It can be done now in not over a half-hour."

Bill readily agreed. In fact, he was ready for anything that promised relief from his suffering, which was so bad that he was considering suicide. The operation was performed with Bill drowsy from medications. Previously, it would have required opening the skin and muscles of the back, but now it was done without making an incision at all. A needle was placed into the area of the spinal cord where the pain pathway ran. The needle was guided into the proper position under the magic of X-ray television. Thus, the neurosurgeon was able to place the fine electrical wire into the pain pathway in the spinal cord that controlled the painful sensations that came from Bill's right leg.

The entire operation only took about twenty-five minutes and was entirely successful as far as relieving the pain. Bill was free of pain for the remaining four months of his life. While it is true that the operation did not add to his life, it did relieve his excruciating pain and made his last months easier. In this respect percutaneous cordotomy, or stereotaxic cordotomy, is indeed a blessing to suffering victims of cancer.

There are many other operations that neurosurgeons can perform to relieve chronic pain. Sometimes a special electrode can be placed over the spinal cord. This remarkable technique was recently popularized by a neurosurgeon named C. Norman Shealy of Wisconsin. Dr. Shealy devised a fine electrode the size of a postage stamp. He places it on the back of the spinal cord where the dorsal (back) columns are located. A fine electrical wire is tunneled under the skin and attached to a stimulator that the patient can press from time to time to send impulses to the spinal cord. These impulses relieve the pain. The principle is similar to the pacemaker, which is attached to the chest of heart patients. The big exception is that the pacemaker is automatic and does not require any stimulation by the patient.

This dorsal column stimulator is an entirely new approach to the relief of pain. It is the exact opposite in action to stereotaxic cordotomy. In the latter case, the nerves are blocked. While this prevents pain impulses from getting through to the brain and relieves the pain, it also removes all sensation, leaving the leg and hip numb. Bill, the cancer patient who received a stereotaxic cordotomy, was more than willing to accept the numbness in exchange for relief from his terrible pain.

Dr. Shealy's work with the dorsal column stimulator has given relief to those patients whose persistent back and leg pains failed to respond to other treatments. It has the advantage that no nerves are cut, and the patient does not feel any numbness as he does when nerves are treated by a stereotaxic cordotomy. But the dorsal column stimulator has no place in treatment of cancer pain.

Psychosurgery

Psychosurgery was popular in the late 1940s and early 1950s, before tranquilizing drugs became available. At that time neurosurgeons hoped to help patients who had severe mental disturbances by disconnecting parts of the frontal lobe of the brain. This is the part of the brain behind the fore-

head that governs thinking and reasoning. Then a neurosurgeon, who had just operated on a mental patient who was
also suffering great pain, noticed that the patient did not
complain of any more pain after the operation.

Later, this same doctor was treating a patient who had
cancer of the breast that was accompanied by extreme pain.
Treatments to relieve the pain were frustrated by the patient's
intensive worry and anxiety. The doctor recalled his previous
case where the brain operation to relieve the patient's mental
anxiety had also appeared to have relieved his pain as well.
With this experience in mind, the doctor deliberately recommended a prefrontal lobotomy to relieve the cancer patient's
pain. The operation he then performed appeared to be successful. Since that time many of these operations have been
performed for patients who have intense pain with associated
anxiety.

More sophisticated techniques of psychosurgery have been
developed in the past twenty years. Dr. Edwin Foltz, a professor of neurosurgery at the University of California at
Irvine, has been popularizing a technique of destroying a part
of the brain known as the cingulum to relieve pain associated
with anxiety. His technique has an advantage over the standard prefrontal lobotomy in that the patient does not become
as confused.

Other surgical techniques to relieve pain include thalamic
surgery. This operation is performed on the thalamus, the
area of the brain that receives and distributes impulses routed
up through the spinal cord by the nerves in the body. This
operation—a thalamotomy—was used in the 1950s and
1960s for relief of the shaking that accompanies Parkinson's
disease prior to the introduction of Levodopa, a drug that
helps control Parkinson's disease in many patients. An exten-
sion of these original techniques now includes deliberate
operations on the thalamus for relief of pain.

The thalamus contains all of the nerve sensations that come into the great computer of the brain, yet paradoxically, neurosurgeons have not been able to relieve pain by disconnecting parts of the thalamus. This is a mystery to us, because this tiny area of the brain contains the termination of all sensations from various parts of the body. Perhaps in the future neurosurgeons will develop the technique of implanting a tiny electrode in the thalamus. Of itself and through a small implanted computer, the electrode could bombard the thalamus with impulses to control pain. This, however, is just speculation on my part.

Acupuncture

Acupuncture, the placing of needles in the body to relieve pain, is rooted in Chinese antiquity. It has been known to the Western world for centuries but has only aroused serious medical attention here within the past two years. This interest came about as a direct result of President Nixon's trip to China in 1971 which opened up an increased exchange of information between our countries. The Chinese reported that they were using acupuncture techniques in connection with major operations, and a great interest developed in these techniques.

Naturally, such a theory did not impress Western medical scientists, who prefer to believe that illness is caused by microbes. However, after reports that acupuncture was being used in place of anesthetics in major operations were verified by Western doctors, this ancient art had to be seriously evaluated.

It is not accurate to say that acupuncture produces anesthesia. More precisely, it produces analgesia or a diminuation of pain. *Anesthesia*, a word introduced by Dr. Oliver Wendell Homes at the end of the nineteenth century, means loss of all feeling. The placement of needles for acupuncture to perform an operation for, say, appendicitis does not render the patient unconscious or totally lacking in feeling of sensation. The early descriptions we received about the use of acupuncture in major operations were interpreted to mean that the patient feels pressure and is aware of what is going on but does not feel pain.

Acupuncture has been tried as a technique to alleviate certain chronic pains. It has been used successfully to control some low back pain, neck sprains, and even sciatic pains. While the Chinese use acupuncture for every type of pain, most American physicians will not use acupuncture without knowing precisely the cause of the pain.

This brings us to the philosophy of Chinese medicine, which also includes pulse diagnosis. The Chinese physician is trained to feel the pulse at the wrist. From this he claims he can diagnose all sorts of disorders of the heart, lungs, liver, kidneys, etc. Of course, the traditional picture of the old family doctor shows him with his hand on a patient's pulse, but the American doctor is checking heartbeat; he is not trying to discover what is wrong with his patient's kidneys.

American physicians, as well as European physicians, have studied the Chinese techniques of pulse diagnosis, but to the best of my knowledge, they have not been able to master it. We prefer to rely on the approved techniques of X-ray diagnosis and laboratory studies to determine the real cause of disease.

For example, suppose you complained of indigestion, nausea, and a severe pain under the right rib cage. In China the doctor might make a diagnosis by feeling your pulse. In the West we would take an X ray to make certain that you did not have a stone in your gall bladder before proceeding with a treatment. We certainly would not use acupuncture as a treatment until after a positive diagnosis was made. We feel that if there is a stone in the gall bladder—as these symptoms suggest—and it is not relieved, then the gall bladder may become inflamed, and an abscess might follow with very serious consequences. Therefore, acupuncture just to relieve pain without getting to the cause, if removable, is not, to our way of thinking, medically sound.

However, acupuncture does have a place in the relief of chronic pain of muscular or neuralgic origins. In my limited experience acupuncture has shown itself capable of helping perhaps one patient in four with this type of pain.

Psychologic Techniques to Relieve Pain

Any person who has suffered pain for a long time and has gone from doctor to doctor will sooner or later be made to feel that both his doctors and his friends think his pain is imagined. A busy doctor may sometimes give this impression to his patient in pain who is on the medical merry-go-round.

The patient is told or made to feel that he is a "crock." This is not a pleasant word. It is the term used by young doctors in large busy hospitals who have to reevaluate patients who have had many operations and still complain of pain. In medical jargon, *crock* is perhaps an abbreviation of a chronic complainer. These same young physicians, when they are older and perhaps have undergone personal suffering and pain, change their attitudes toward chronic pain sufferers.

It is in conditions like this that psychologic techniques are most important. Anyone who suffers chronic or long enduring pain must have a high degree of nervousness and anxiety associated with it.

I recall a personal experience in which I had been suffering chest pains that would not clear up. Even though I am a doctor and despite negative X rays of my lungs, I was still worried and became quite nervous over the pain. Ask anyone who has had operations for a slipped disc and failed to improve why he has become irrritable, anxious, and worried.

Pain, in addition to the suffering that it produces, causes us to withdraw from the activities of everyday life. After a while we spend our lives just thinking of the pain. Day after day we have to live with it, knowing there is no magic relief in sight. This is a condition few of us can face with a pleasant smile.

When people get into this frame of mind, the techniques of the psychologist and psychiatrist are most helpful. First, the doctor must understand that the patient's associated anxiety is based on reality and is not imagined. This understanding goes a long way to help the patient accept the pain. Secondly, the patient must be made to understand that the pain itself will not destroy him but that the morbid and anxious thoughts about the pain can do so. This helps him understand that even though something positive cannot be done for him at this time, his attitude toward his condition can make his situation worse. Just a change of attitude can make a definite improvement.

Sometimes pain is associated with a high degree of resentment and anger. There is bitterness because we must suffer, while others are spared our agony. Such thoughts add anxiety and strain, which in turn materially affect our condition. The pain is real enough, but bitter resentment is something else. Doctors may not be able to lessen the real pain, but a change in the patient's attitude toward his pain and his circumstances can lessen his total pain. Control of your emotional reaction to pain is a partial painkiller in itself. Since this emotional reaction is a product of the mind and the emotions, it cannot be helped by medicine. It must come from the mind of the patient, guided by sympathetic and understanding help from someone who understands this perfectly natural reaction.

When the Good Life Turns Bad

Finally, there are the patients whom we can classify as "pain losers." These are people who have been materially, spiritually, and socially fortunate in life. They always had good reason to believe that life was going their way, and they never dreamed that things would ever be any different.

Then, suddenly, they find themselves the victims of chronic pains that throb and beat against their nerves night and day. Possibly the unexpected change came from a slipped disc or an injury to the low back so that the pain encompasses the back and a leg.

The sweet life has now turned sour. In addition to the constant agony, this type of pain is often associated with loss of work, loss of income, and even court litigation. Now the medical merry-go-round starts turning. The patient's life becomes a ceaseless series of visits to doctors' offices. These visits may be to seek relief from his agony or they may be ordered by insurance companies. Resentment builds up. You feel that the insurance company, in forcing you to see company doctors, is trying to get out of paying you. If litigation is involved, you may feel that doctors for the insurance company are trying to rob you of what you have coming to you. Whether there is any real basis for these beliefs is not important. They exist and must be taken into account by the doctor if he hopes to help his patient.

All this endless parade from one doctor to another keeps the patient's mind focused constantly upon his infirmity. He builds resentment to an exploding point instead of learning to bear his trouble as best he can.

It is only natural for this type of patient to turn the full measure of his resentment, anger, and hostility toward his own doctor as well. He has failed him. This is untrue, of course. Doctors do care. But it is very difficult to convince a suffering patient and keep him from developing an attitude of "I'm a loser. What's the use? Life's passing me by."

In some cases the psychiatrist discovers that the patient is using his pain as an excuse to keep from making an effort to help himself. This is much like the accident-prone person who is always getting into minor accidents to avoid the responsibilities of life. This defense mechanism is not difficult to understand. All of us recall times in our childhood when we pleaded a tummy ache to avoid going to school.

Pain then is not only a product of the physical disorder that causes it but also is modified by our emotional reactions to the discomfort. The final pain we feel is the sum of these two products. *Therefore, pain is always an individual sensation that has a different meaning to each of us.* This individual reaction permits some people to tolerate a large amount of pain and continue to work through it. Artists, for example, are often sensitive, high-strung individuals. I know of a musician who sometimes gives his best performances while suffering the most terrible migraine headaches. After his performance he often collapses from nausea and head pain, but during the two hours he is playing the violin he is able to rise above his pain. There are many examples of this sort of thing. And each of us, I am sure, can remember some emergency when we completely forgot our own problems in a rush to help others.

Conditioned Reflexes

Psychological techniques to control pain can also make use of conditioned reflexes. Fifty years ago Ivan Pavlov showed that a dog could be trained to salivate in response to the sound of a bell. Similar control of animal reflexes has been subsequently shown in many ways by other investigators. From these experiments it is reasonable to conclude that a person can be conditioned to accept certain amounts of pain as something perfectly natural.

Dr. Wilbert Fordyce, in the May 1973 issue of *Post-Graduate Medicine*, demonstrated that a knowledge of conditioned reflexes or operant conditioning can help many patients with chronic pains. Dr. Fordyce argues that the usual response to pain—screaming, asking for help, or calling a physician—may work in the beginning when initial pain is severe. As the pain becomes longstanding, the same type of behavioral response—along with grimaces and holding the back (in the case of low back pain)—becomes just a learned or behavioral response. Like the dog who slobbers at the sound of a bell, we have conditioned ourselves to respond to a twinge of pain in a reflex pattern.

Unfortunately, physicians may label such patients as having psychogenic pain or being hysterical. When such patients are examined by psychiatrists or psychologists and the hysterical component is not found, then the treating physician becomes disturbed himself. This is why, Dr. Fordyce points out, there is a low rate of success with psychotherapy in treating chronic pain patients. His argument that some patients develop a pain habit is a good one. Each time the patient complains of pain to free himself from an unpleasant duty, he is reenforcing his complaint.

Some patients use their pain to get attention. Children are good at this. And we sometimes see housewives who get attention from their husbands when they have a headache or back trouble and repeat their complaints every time they feel deprived of attention. What such a wife does not understand is that the sympathy she elicited in the beginning may wear off with time. Anything constantly repeated loses its effectiveness, and her husband will eventually become tired and disgusted at her constant complaints. What started out as a good thing for her will later on become a burden.

Often elderly people learn that they only get attention when they are suffering. Children are then more solicitous about calling them. Neighbors, too, are helpful. Friends remember them.

Summary

Research into the psychological aspects of pain teaches us that there are advantages in pain for certain types of people. It brings them attention, affection, and freedom from unpleasant activity.

The basic techniques for helping relieve chronic pain are:
• complete physical examination, including an evaluation by specialists;
• skillful use of drugs, other than aspirin, to control pain;
• physical techniques of massage, ultrasound, and hydrotherapy;
• nerve surgery to give permanent relief of pain, including the newer technique of stereotaxic cordotomy;
• acupuncture; and
• psychotherapy and psychological techniques.

6

RHEUMATISM AND ARTHRITIS AS CAUSES OF CHRONIC PAIN

Barbara was anxiously waiting to see me. She complained of severe pain and tingling in her fingers. She told me that for the past several months she would awaken in the very early morning with this severe pain and tingling.

My examination found only very tender fingers, especially in the joints of her hand, and nothing more. A complete neurologic examination followed. It showed that she still had good power in her hands. She appreciated pin pricks in both hands and in all her fingers. This was encouraging, for I could find nothing that would explain her pain as neuritis—inflammation—of a nerve to the hand, or an irritation of the nerves as they left her neck.

Barbara was a commercial artist, married to Tim, a free-lance producer of documentary motion pictures. During their early years together they had been too busy to have children. But now at thirty-one she wanted a child. She and Tim had not been successful in having one. Under the circumstances it was logical to suspect a possible emotional stimulus to at least part of her pain. As it happened, she did have an emotional problem. However, it stemmed from her pain rather than being a contributory cause of it. She suddenly revealed her feeling as we were going over the results of her initial tests.

"Doctor!" she burst out. Her voice, the strained look on her face, and the tension in her body clearly revealed the depth of her emotional state.

"Did you know that my mother suffers from severe arthritis?" she asked. "I'm sure that I've inherited the same thing. I'm going to be a cripple!"

"Well," I said, speaking as gently as I could, "*you* may be sure, but I'm not and I'm the doctor. There's no cause yet to push the panic button."

"You'd get panicky too if you found yourself becoming a cripple at thirty-one like I am!" she cried fiercely.

"Again, let me say, don't push the panic button until you have something to panic about," I replied. "You are not a cripple and I don't think you are going to become one. Now listen carefully to me. . . ."

I went on to tell her the full results of my tests. She did not have a ruptured disc pressing on the nerves of her upper limbs. There was no compression by an abnormal rib or anything else that might indicate a definite cause for Barbara's severe pain.

I did agree that she might have arthritis, but there was no cause for her extreme alarm. Arthritis takes many forms. I wanted my diagnosis checked out by a specialist. So I sent her to a rheumatologist—a specialist in diseases of the joints. His report indicated an early case of *rheumatoid arthritis*—a type that causes severe swelling of the joints. She was advised to have a series of tests and X rays to verify the diagnosis. One of the blood tests, called the sedimentation rate, confirmed that she probably had rheumatoid arthritis.

Her treatment consisted of a maximum amount of rest, interspersed with periods of exercises to keep her joints from stiffening. Fortunately, there was no indication of associated problems of her heart or blood. Her pain was controlled by heavy doses of an aspirin substitute, which did not irritate her stomach. In about three weeks she was over the roughest period of her discomfort.

Later, Barbara became pregnant and most of her symptoms subsided. This is not unusual in patients with rheumatoid arthritis.

Lessons to Be Learned from Barbara's Case

The first lesson we have to pass on to patients with rheumatoid arthritis is that they are not suffering from a fatal disease. It is one that has its ups and downs, however. Painkillers and rest are the most important treatments, and, of course, the right kind of exercise to prevent stiffening of the joints. Certain types of diets, living in drier climates, and wearing copper bracelets—to name some suggested aids to the arthritic—do *not* help. As for the recent fascination with acupuncture as a means of controlling arthritic pain, it does no more than just that—control pain in occasional cases. Acupuncture does not get to the source of the arthritic trouble.

Some Facts about Arthritis

The term arthritis is not a good one. Arthritis means an inflammation of a joint. The first syllable refers to a joint, and the *itis* means inflammation.

Inflammation refers to a reaction of our tissues to an irritation, caused either by an injury or by bacterial invasion of a part of the body. Some of its main signs are pain, swelling, redness, heat, and disturbed function. So we speak of tonsillitis, colitis, and appendicitis all in the same breath, to indicate by the suffix *itis* that there is an inflammation of a particular part of the body. The *itis* does not mean that we have a specific cause we can isolate, such as a particular microbe. It is a general term to identify a condition.

Rheumatism is an old term and is still used for arthritis. In fact, we do not speak of an arthritis specialist as much as we say a rheumatologist. The official designation of the class of this disease today is rheumatology. However, most doctors prefer to say arthritis.

We do not know the cause of arthritis. We know what it is: an inflammation of a joint. But except in a few cases we do not know the source of this inflammation. Severe inflammation of an arthritic type can be seen in some gonorrhea cases. Tuberculosis is another example where joints can be affected. Syphilis can also cause a deformity of a joint. This condition is known as Charcot's joint, after a famous French physician who first described it.

Types of Arthritis

There are a number of different types of arthritis. The following are the most common types.

RHEUMATOID

This is the most severe type. It occurs more frequently in women than in men, reaching a peak incidence between the ages of thirty-five and forty. It is associated with severe swelling and pain in the joint. When it affects the hands, as in Barbara's case, it involves the more proximal joints (those at the point of an attachment of a limb) rather than the fingertips. Severe fatigue and anemia are generally associated with rheumatoid arthritis attacks. The blood test known as the sedimentation rate can show abnormality.

DEGENERATIVE JOINT DISEASE

It is frightening to the average person to be told that he has something that is degenerative, but the medical name *hypertrophic osteoarthritis* is hardly an improvement. This heavy expression actually indicates very little other than a thickening of the joint ends. This is due to a laying down of bone at the joint, or—as it is often popularly described—as a buildup of calcium at the joint.

To hear the word degenerative applied to themselves can often be a traumatic shock to patients. I remember very well the case of Robert, a fifty-five-year-old stockbroker. He was suffering from chronic backaches and leg pains and had been told that he needed an operation on his back. He came to me for a neurosurgical opinion before submitting to the operation. My examination showed him to be flabby and somewhat potbellied. This plus total baldness and worry made Robert look much older than his fifty-five years.

It was obvious that he was more worried than his condition warranted. But before I could make inquiries to probe the state of his mind, he suddenly blurted out the cause of his worry. His previous doctor had told him that his trouble was degenerative arthritis. "I guess I'm just rotting away," he said, his forlorn face reflecting his misery.

"Why do you say that, Bob?" I asked.

"The other doctor told me I have a degenerative disc."

"Didn't you ask him what that meant?" I replied.

"I didn't have to ask," he said. "I know what degenerative means. After all, I did go to school once."

"Then your school should have taught you that the same word has many meaning sometimes," I replied. "Degenerative, applied to a person's character, certainly is something to disturb someone. But degenerative applied to arthritis simply means normal wear and tear. It happens to all of us. To me as well as to you."

"You really mean it?" he asked doubtfully. "You're not just trying to make me feel good."

I assured him that I thought a doctor's job was to make people feel good and that I certainly hoped that I would do so in his case. However, I added, he had no cause for alarm. His examination showed that there was no need for him to rush into an operation (laminectomy). His leg pain was not severe, and I thought that he would respond to a program of exercises and weight loss. And, I am pleased to say, he did respond.

Unfortunately, the term *degenerative arthritis* is commonplace among physicians. I personally avoid it, because it always arouses needless fears in patients, and for a very good reason: It sounds like something terrible but is as natural as graying hair, falling teeth, hardening of the arteries—all natural outcomes of living.

This type of arthritis commonly occurs in people over forty. But only a small percent of us with *osteoarthritis* (degenerative joint disease) have associated pain. In a typical case it affects the fingers. There can be swelling and deformity at the last (distal) joint of the finger. There will be little bulbous thickenings on either side of the joint. These are call Heberden's nodes after the British physician who first described them years ago. They make a woman's hands look less dainty but do not, of themselves, deform the joint or stiffen it.

GOUTY ARTHRITIS

Gout is a specific type of joint disease that has a tendency to affect the big toe, although gouty arthritis can affect many other joints as well. It is seen more frequently in men than in women. An attack can bring swelling and severe pain to the big toe, making walking impossible.

In former times, gout was considered the hallmark of the wealthy, who were supposed to have eaten a hearty diet of kidneys or food rich in purines. The diagnosis of gout is easy to make, because during the severe, acute pain an elevation of uric acid may occur in the blood. Another proof of the diagnosis is response of the patient to a drug known as colchicine. If the gout symptoms subside in one week's use, then the diagnosis is almost certain.

MISCELLANEOUS ARTHRITIS AND RHEUMATOLOGIC DISORDERS

Lumped into this group are a variety of such ailments as tennis elbow, housemaid's knee, and the traumatic arthritis that follows repeated injuries to the neck, as in whiplash injuries, which are so common in automobile collisions.

How to Help Yourself Manage Severe Arthritic Pain

Since easily ten million Americans have some form of arthritic pain, the control of this type of discomfort becomes a major medical problem and one that promises tremendous benefit to humanity. It has been estimated that millions of work hours are lost annually because of arthritis, in addition to the hours, days, and years of agony suffered by those who have the disease.

It is quite possible, of course, that this diagnosis is overworked. Hardly a doctor in a busy practice fails to make this diagnosis in a large percentage of his patients who come to him with complaints of pain in the neck or low back regions. I suppose most of us have heard at one time or another a doctor tell us, "You have a touch of arthritis in your neck." Or it may have been in your back or legs or hands. Some of these many minor arthritic diagnoses may have been only sprains and muscle strains that produce similar symptoms.

In controlling arthritic pain, the following are very practical points to remember:

• Once your doctor makes the diagnosis of arthritis, you, the patient, must take over and care for yourself. You are much like the diabetic who has to control his diet and even learn to check urine for sugar content.

• Pain is the enemy in arthritis. It can be conquered by the use of aspirin and its substitutes.

• You must also learn to use physical measures, such as warm baths, hot packs, and exercises.

• You must not be discouraged by fatigue. You must consider it a signal that you should allow more rest to your joints. It is better to work in short spells, forcing yourself to rest and then to exercise. In other words, instead of planning to work three or four hours at a time, you should settle for one hour's work and then take a fifteen minute rest period before starting again.

• Discouragement and pushing the panic button are among your greatest enemies. You must develop confidence in yourself and in your ability to recover.

• Your mental state is extremely important. Rheumatoid arthritis has been associated with acute psychological injury. The sudden death of a loved one or severe financial reverses can precipitate severe arthritis. It is important, therefore, to recognize this and to develop an attitude of cheerfulness toward your infirmity. Develop a positive outlook toward life and, if necessary, even accept the reality of your limitations. Sometimes some practical psychotherapy, given by your doctor, will go a long way toward helping you overcome your periods of pain and their accompanying depression.

• Don't believe in any miracle drug for arthritis. There is no single drug at present that will control this condition.

• You must have strong confidence in your ability to see your condition through, even though it may last a long time—maybe even a lifetime. There will be ups and downs in your condition that only you can control.

Some Questions about Pain in Arthritis

QUESTION: Will I die from the pain of my arthritis?

ANSWER: No one ever dies from pain in the joints. I have seen some patients with severe facial pain of trigeminal neuralgia go so far as to try suicide to escape their excruciating pain. But in chronic arthritis the pain itself will not cause a patient to want to kill himself.

QUESTION: What can I do about the pain?

ANSWER: You can do much for the pain, as I have already described. But most of all you must have a regular routine of exercise. This must be carried out even though you may not feel like doing it. Exercises need not and should not be vigorous.

For example, let us suppose that you have a pain in your neck. The first hour in the morning is generally the worst. You take a few aspirin to help you. Do not hesitate to apply hot moist packs to your neck as well. Then, with heat still in your muscles, force yourself to rotate your head from side to side. This can be done by placing a pillow under your shoulders and bending your head backward. Then, gently rotate your neck from side to side. You may prefer to do this in a chair, and you can roll your head around.

If the pain is in your hip, then it is easy to sit on the side of a table and swing your hip backward and forward. Your doctor can show you a good routine of exercises. Or you can obtain a book giving pictures and descriptions of these exercises by writing to the Arthritis and Rheumatism Foundation, 10 Columbus Circle, New York City, New York 10019.

QUESTION: Will I be crippled for life or totally invalided by my arthritis?

ANSWER: This question is uppermost in the minds of every arthritis patient. It is a question steeped in deep emotion, and unless it is resolved in the patient's mind, it can greatly hinder his or her progress. Barbara, whose case history we recounted earlier, is an example. She was so certain that she faced a future as a cripple that she built up strains and tensions that actually made her condition worse than it should have been. If she had not cleansed her mind of her morbid fears, there is a good chance that she might have become a cripple.

Let me say this in all sincerity to those who suffer from arthritis: If you follow a careful routine to control the pain, force yourself to move, and have confidence that you will not become a cripple, then the chances are very small that this will happen to you.

Most arthritic patients who have become crippled are those who have neglected themselves from the start or who have failed to follow the advice of their doctors. They literally allow their joints to freeze into a crippled state. You must believe that you will not be crippled.

QUESTION: Can I still lead a useful life, even with arthritis?

ANSWER: Let's say that the worst that happens is that you are forced to use a wheelchair to get around from time to time. You can still overcome your difficulties. You may remember the famous actor Lionel Barrymore. In his last years he was confined to a wheelchair. Yet he never left the screen. He continued to delight millions who came to see the Dr. Kildare and Dr. Gillespie pictures in which he appeared despite his infirmity. In not letting his condition force him into inactivity, Barrymore surely added years to his life and brought pleasure to those who admired his acting skill.

INJECTIONS INTO JOINTS

When cortisone was first derived, it became available in liquid form as hydrocortisone for injections into painful joints. During the acute phase of pain and swelling of arthritic joints, this type of treatment, when given by a specialist, has proven to be a great benefit in many cases.

But cortisone will not help the degenerative type of arthritis, because this is a problem of wear and tear—a part of the life process. So do not expect a magical return for deformed joints from this type of treatment. But anyone who has had an injection of cortisone into a painful bursa (the pouchlike cavity between the joints) or into a painful tennis-type elbow has become grateful.

WHAT ABOUT SURGERY?

There is no specific operation for arthritis. Sometimes a joint becomes so badly crippled that it must be replaced by an artificial joint. The hip joint and the knee are the commonest operations of this type. Such joint surgery is no longer experimental and is routinely performed. It has proven to be a great help in controlling pain, especially in the hip and knee.

Other operations, such as those to overcome deformity of fingers and knuckles, must be considered with great caution. As a neurosurgeon, I have performed operations on the cervical (neck) and lower spine to relieve crippling pain symptoms when patients experienced excess pressure on nerve roots.

In this type of surgery, called a laminectomy, pressure from the nerve roots is removed. This operation in no way alters the course of the arthritis itself. It is recommended only for the control of extreme discomfort or chronic pain in the arms and legs.

MEDICATIONS OR DRUGS

I keep repeating the value of aspirin for arthritic relief. This is because salicylates, of which aspirin is the commonest type, still make up the main drug used to relieve the acute pain and suffering of this disease. All other drugs are combinations of chemicals similar to salicylates. Unfortunately, excessive aspirin does cause stomach irritation and even bleeding in some patients. A long-acting coated aspirin has been developed to eliminate this undesirable side effect. For the same reason, newer compounds such as Tylenol and similar ones with less toxic ingredients are used for relief of arthritis pain and discomfort.

Other drugs like the gold salts and the wonder drug cortisone and its derivatives have been used in some arthritics. Cortisone was originally derived from animal adrenal glands but now can be synthetically prepared.

However, it is important to remember that there is no specific medication to cure arthritis the way quinine, for example, subdues the symptoms of malaria. Most patients who try the drug route in search of arthritic pain relief sooner or later give it up. In the end they come back to simple aspirin as the best of them all. Of course, no drug should be used without the continued supervision of your doctor.

WHAT ABOUT ACUPUNCTURE FOR ARTHRITIS PAIN RELIEF?

There have been many reports recently of the efficacy of acupuncture to overcome painful joints associated with arthritis. A recent study, trying to prove or disprove the value of acupuncture, revealed that patients with painful, swollen knees were relieved of pain for a period of time when treated by acupuncture.

This temporary relief of pain compared favorably with the injection of hydrocortisone injections into the knee joint. But there was one big difference: The cortisone injection relieved the pain but also controlled the swelling associated with the arthritic knee. Acupuncture relieved the pain but did not control the swelling.

It would appear from this study that acupuncture—at least in the treatment of this particular type of arthritis—is of value as a painkiller only. It does not provide a specific cure. But as a painkiller, acupuncture will find greater use in many patients who have severe pain of arthritis.

Some Do's and Don'ts for Arthritis

• Consult a good family physician and if you have trouble finding one, write to the American Board of Family Medicine or the Academy of General Practice, Volker Boulevard at Brookside Boulevard, Kansas City, Missouri, for the name of a good physician in your area. Any well-trained family physician can direct your care. If he thinks you need a specialist of any type, let him direct you, rather than doing it yourself.

• Maintain a program of hopeful treatment. Eat a full diet with plenty of minerals and vitamins.

• Be religious about performing a steady range of exercises. This will insure that your joints do not stiffen or rust out. As an old neurologist friend of mine, Louis Doshay, used to tell his patients with Parkinson's disease, "running water never freezes." By this he meant that you must keep exercising to maintain life in your joints. Your doctor can send you to a good physical therapist who can teach you the type of exercises you need. Or, as mentioned before, you can send for the booklet of exercises published by the American Rheumatism and Arthritis Foundation. The value of exercises to prevent your "running water from freezing" cannot be overemphasized and is worth constantly repeating.

• Heat is one of the oldest and most useful of all types of therapy. However, you should be careful in its use, whether it be moist heat or dry heat. The use of heat should be done under the guidance of your physician. Patients treating themselves have been know to sustain serious burns from the use of heat. Sometimes, due to lack of skin sensitivity or the depth of the basic pain that overshadows that of the skin, a patient has burned himself without being aware of it.

• Remember you can lead a useful life even though you have a chronic pain of arthritis, if you make up your mind that you can be helped and that your pain is something to be relieved.

• Don't be suckered by cure-alls. There are more arthritis quacks to take the money of the ten million or more arthritic sufferers than you can imagine. Only the diet faddists are second to the arthritic faddists.

• Don't expect trips to expensive spas to help your condition. A dry warm climate is easier to live in, but it does not affect the course of arthritis.

• Don't waste money on fancy exercise machines. All the exercises you need can be prescribed by your doctor.

• Don't use sagging mattresses, soft chairs, sloppy posture, and improperly fitting shoes. They all put strain and tension on your body and spine.

• Don't panic—this above all. If your doctor tells you that you have degenerative arthritis, it does not mean that you are falling apart. *Degenerative* is a bad term, but we use it. Remember that it only means wear and tear—the normal process of living.

There are many famous people who have contributed greatly to the world despite suffering the ravages of arthritis.

The famous French painter Pierre Auguste Renoir was crippled by arthritis in his last years. Still he refused to give up his painting, which had meant so much to him all through his long life. He had himself strapped into a chair, and special holders on his crippled fingers held his brushes so that he could still paint. He continued to work up to the time of his death. Observe a Renoir with all its scintillating color and youthful beauty to remind you that life can still be beautiful and productive even though you are suffering.

7

HEADACHES, MIGRAINES, AND OTHER HEAD PAINS

Larry was a hard-driving, get-things-done attorney. A man in his late forties, he had fought his way to the top of his profession and intended to stay there. And his way of staying on top was to work night and day. He liked to brag that he thrived on work and was never sick a day in his life. In making such a statement, he ignored the migraine headaches that had been part of his life since his college days. They had become a way of life with him. He gulped down some aspirin when they came on and went about his business.

Then, one day, his headaches took a turn for the worse. He began going to bed with a severely pounding head. Once or twice during the night he had to get up and take some aspirin compound for relief. The next morning he would stumble out of bed bleary-eyed from lack of sleep and wondering how he could possibly get through the important trial scheduled for court that day. He felt dizzy when he tried to shave. He swallowed some more aspirin, drank some black coffee, and hurried off to court without a full breakfast. Despite his slight dizziness and nausea, he managed to win most of his cases.

He had once said that the secret of his success in life was that he could look at himself objectively. Most people cannot. Thus, he was able to evaluate his faults as well as his virtues and profit from both. Now he tried to look at his condition just as objectively. As a lawyer he applied logic and decided that his headaches were due to tension. He was in the middle of a series of extremely important lawsuits that involved very large sums of money. The outcome of these cases not only meant a lot to Larry's client—a large corporation—but to himself as well. He objectively admitted that he might be working too hard but excused himself on the grounds that it was necessary to further his career. They will go away when these cases are over, he assured himself.

But they did not go away. The headaches got progressively worse. After a few weeks of increasing agony, Larry finally gave in and called his family physician. The doctor was an old friend who had known Larry since they were undergraduates together.

"So you're having another of your migraine attacks, Larry," the doctor said when the lawyer came to see him one afternoon.

"It's more than a headache this time," Larry said, pressing the palms of his hands against his aching temples. "I feel like fifty judges are inside my head, and all are banging their gavels on my nerves at the same time."

"That bad, huh?" the doctor said, frowning slightly as he observed the dark circles under Larry's eyes and the haggard lines in his face.

"They are the worst I've ever had," Larry replied. "And, they have stayed on the longest. I've been in misery for the past two weeks. I thought it was just tension because I was bogged down in some very important cases. I was sure the headaches would go away when the trials were over."

"That's what *you* thought," the doctor replied rather caustically. "But what *I* thought was that we had an agreement. I'd do your doctoring and you'd do my lawyering and we'd both stay out of the other's profession."

"Well, I'm here now," Larry said lamely. "Start doctoring."

"Better late then never, I guess. Now I know you've had migraines sinces you were eighteen. What makes this one different from all the others?"

"The main thing that makes it different is that it hurts more," Larry replied. "And most of the time I've been able to shake off my headaches with a few aspirin and a little sleep."

The doctor then checked Larry's blood pressure and made some neurologic tests. He looked into Larry's eyes with the ophthalmoscope to observe the blood vessels and nerve in the back of the eye, which was normal. The patient's blood pressure was elevated slightly but was not abnormally high. There were no changes in Larry's reflexes.

"There doesn't *seem* to be anything wrong," the doctor admitted reluctantly. "Maybe you are just having a migraine storm. Anyway, here's a prescription for a little stronger medication. If the headaches don't respond to it in forty-eight hours, then check in with me again."

Still the doctor was dissatisfied. Larry's migraine headaches were not following their normal pattern. This worried him. As his patient and friend was dressing, the doctor asked abruptly: "Larry, are you sure that you have told me everything about these headaches? Are you sure that you haven't had some disturbance or other pains or bumps or something?"

"Nothing," Larry said. "I did get a bump on the handball court, but it was nothing."

"Tell me about it anyway," the doctor said.

"Oh, I banged my head into the side of the court about three weeks ago," Larry replied. "I fell and my partner had to pick me up. I was dazed for a couple of minutes, but it cleared up and I went on to win the game. It was nothing."

"I'm not so sure about that," the doctor insisted. "This might be the source of your headaches."

"No, no! That's ridiculous. I didn't feel a thing the next day. These headaches didn't start for a week after that."

"Maybe so," the doctor replied. "Anyway, take this medicine tonight, and if the pain is worse tomorrow, I want you to see a specialist."

He wrote a name and address on a card and gave it to Larry. The pain was worse the next morning. In fact, it was almost unbearable. Larry did see the neurologic specialist that his family doctor had recommended. More neurologic tests were made, with the same results obtained by the family physician. Then, although Larry complained that it was a waste of time, the specialist insisted that Larry have some special tests to rule out any suggestion that the blow on his head had anything to do with his increased head pains.

More because he felt too bad to argue than his belief that the tests would prove anything, Larry entered the hospital for a few days of tests. He rather welcomed it, for he hoped that the rest would cure the tension that he still blamed for his trouble.

Instead, he was stunned when his doctors told him that one of the tests, a brain scan, showed an abnormal area over the right side of his head. This was strongly indicative of a subdural hematoma, which they defined as a blood clot on the brain. With this evidence to guide them, his doctors began new probing. Larry recalled that he had been feeling excessively sleepy lately. This was not his accustomed attitude, but he had attributed it to sleeplessness caused by his night pain. The sleepiness fitted in with the diagnosis of a blood clot on his brain.

The neurologic specialist then had a special cerebral arteriogram made of Larry's brain by injecting a dye into the carotid (neck) blood vessels that supply the brain. The dye, being more opaque to X rays, allows better visualization of the blood vessels in the brain. Any displacement of a blood vessel due to pressure of a blood clot can then be detected from the X rays. The resulting X rays proved this to be true in Larry's case. Once the diagnosis was confirmed, Larry was cured by a relatively safe craniotomy—an operation to drain off the blood.

Lessons to Be Learned from Larry's Case

One of the basic lessons to learn from Larry's case is that a person is a poor judge of his own condition. Twice Larry guessed wrong about his symptoms, which caused him to put off seeking medical attention. His first diagnostic mistake was to assume that his headaches were the result of tension instead of the fall he had taken on the handball court. His second major self-diagnostic error was mistaking the sleepiness as being cause by lack of sleep, when it was actually due to pressure of the blood clot.

Larry might have been right in his self-diagnosis, considering his history of migraine headaches, if his new flurry of head pain had followed the pattern of the first. But these new headaches were different in character. You must always be aware that if your headaches change in character, then something more is happening than usual. This "something" must be investigated. In Larry's case, further delay of proper treatment could have placed him in a very serious condition. The longer you delay treatment, the more difficult the treatment becomes and the less chance you have for an easy recovery.

A subdural hematoma (blood clot), such as Larry experienced, is not a common cause of headaches. The presence of a blood clot or a tumor makes up hardly 5 percent of all headaches. Most headaches, as we will learn later, are due to emotional tension. I use this case as an example despite its comparative rarity, because it shows so well the need for thoroughness in any examination of a sufferer of chronic headaches. This thoroughness applies both to the medical examinations themselves and to the patient in recounting his symptoms to the doctor.

Commonest Types of Headaches

The most common types of headaches can be divided into the following categories:

EMOTIONAL TENSION

This is the kind of headache all of us get at one time or another. It starts many times with a tight feeling in the back of the head. The pain then spreads forward over the top of the head and across the eyes.

We call it an emotional tension headache because it is associated with either an awareness of chronic emotional tension or a sensation of nervousness that will not go away. Anyone who works under pressure or who is exposed to the everyday disease of boredom on the job finds himself in conflict with life as he wants and gets it. In some of us this can set off emotional tension headaches.

This reaction to unpleasantness can take varied forms. Your friend at the desk across the aisle may suffer from recurrent indigestion. Another person may have periods of diarrhea due to colitis. We call these reactions *psychosomatic disturbances*, and the form that they take depends upon the emotional makeup of the individual.

MIGRAINE

About 5 to 10 percent of all headaches fall into the category of migraine. The word is French in origin, but the same spelling is used in English. It means nothing more than a headache that is confined to one half of the head.

A typical migraine attack is often seen in patients who are compulsive about their work or life-styles. The well-dressed, neat blonde who is always so fussy about her appearance may be a target for migraine. These people are artistic and quietly aggressive but hold back their aggression and develop resentment.

A typical attack may start out with a vague feeling of un-easiness. This is followed by a rapid development of throbbing pain in the temple. There may be a shooting sen-sation behind the eye. In certain cases there may be blurring of vision or a zig zag explosion of lights from one side of the visual field. This condition is known as *scintillating scotoma* (blindness). The attack may become so violent over one-half of the head that the patient's neck muscles feel extremely ten-der. At this point the patient may feel severe nausea and even vomit. Bright lights become intolerable to him or her and only sleeping it off will break up the attack.

HEADACHES CAUSED BY SINUS AND EYE TROUBLES

This type of headache has been overrated. Sinus troubles at one time were thought to be a common cause of head-aches. Even disturbances of the eyes were thought to be associated with many head pains. However, when there is a blurring of vision, double vision, or blindness in one part of the visual field associated with chronic headaches, the problem is not coming from the eye. It is coming from inside the head and should be checked into carefully.

Of course, when a person has strong astigmatism (inability of the eye to focus vertical and horizontal lines at the same time), headaches may develop from this condition. When in doubt, you should check with your eye doctor for a complete examination. Glaucoma is another pain in the eye itself. I am not speaking of purely eye disorders that are confined to the eye but to those that spread over the entire head.

Sinuses sometimes cause headaches when they are blocked by severe head colds. But this is a type of headache that is easily detected from the general cold condition, the position of the pain, and the stopped up nostrils.

HEADACHE FOLLOWING A HEAD INJURY OR WHIPLASH

Anyone who has had a blow on the head knows that it hurts. This hurt is due to a jarring of the structures inside the head as well as to tearing or straining of muscles in the back of the head. Why certain people will persist in having head pains long after an injury is still something we cannot clearly explain. But when a headache persists for many weeks after an injury, then you should be suspicious of something more than just the normal jar and strain. Larry's case is a good example of a complication that can follow a head injury.

The so-called whiplash injury, where the head snaps forward and then back again, can be a cause of persistent headaches. These are generally the results of tearing of the muscles in the back of the neck. Automobile collision accidents are a very common source of these whiplash injuries, although they can occur in sports, home injuries, and elsewhere.

MISCELLANEOUS CAUSES OF HEADACHE

About 5 to 8 percent of headaches come from various causes, such as subdural hematoma, as in Larry's case, or brain tumors. Another very important miscellaneous cause of headache is a ruptured blood vessel. An example of this is the famous case of the actress Patricia Neal.

Ruptured blood vessels usually announce their presence with a headache that is literally "out of this world." But it is confined to the back of the neck. It then spreads forward and almost always is associated with a sense of nausea, vomiting, and near collapse. This condition naturally causes a patient extreme apprehension and is always a serious matter.

A patient with such severe headache and pain in the back of the neck should be rushed to a hospital. There the diagnosis can be quickly made by a spinal fluid examination, which will reveal bloody fluid if the cause is a ruptured blood vessel in the brain. Doctors call this a *subarachnoid hemorrhage.*

How to Help Your Doctor Discover the Cause of Your Headaches

Let us suppose that you are suffering from chronic headaches. By this I mean a headache that lingers on for weeks, or one that keeps recurring with regularity. You have tried all the drugs on the market without any notable success. You are now concerned, because the headache will not go away and worry is adding its own complications to your condition.

First of all, if you find yourself in this condition, let me reassure you that the chances are in your favor that there is nothing seriously wrong. Large studies of patients with headaches, done by Harold Wolff of Cornell University, Arnold P. Friedman of Montefiore Hospital, New York, and other investigators, have shown that the vast majority of common headaches—at least 90 percent—are associated with emotional tension. This means that nine times out of ten your headache is something that can be helped.

Another 7 or 8 percent of headaches are migraine. Again, this is not a serious condition, although it can drive you crazy with its periodic disability. This leaves only about 3 percent to make up the really serious classes of headaches, such as subdural hematoma or a ruptured intracranial aneurysm, as in the case of Patricia Neal.

In other words, from 95 to 97 percent of the time your headache is not associated with a serious disorder that can cripple you or take your life.

One of the best ways to help your doctor discover the causes of your headaches is to begin to make yourself an analysis checklist.

Checklist for the Headache Sufferer

1. *List the pattern of your headache.* Are they work-related? Or related to the time of day? Are they aggravated by foods, alcohol, or drugs? Are they aggravated by medicines you may be taking for arthritis or high blood pressure? What you are trying to establish here is whether the headaches occur after any regular activity, duty, or frustration.

2. *Does your family have a history of headaches?* Migraine is notorious for running in families. Many times the mother may pass along this tendency to her sons. It is important for your doctor to know if this tendency runs in your family.

3. *Have you had any head injuries, even trivial ones?* This is extremely important. Even those that you are prone to dismiss should be reported to your doctor. Let him decide if they are unimportant. The case of Larry's fall on the handball court is a graphic example of a "trivial" head injury that developed into something that could have been fatal.

4. *Do you have blurring vision or double vision along with your headaches?*

5. *Do you have any dizziness or vertigo?*

6. *Do you get any relief of your headache from simple aspirin or other drugs or from sleeping in a dark room?*

The answers to these questions can give your doctor important clues to the possible source of your trouble. They can also save him important time by eliminating unprofitable lines of examination. You should come to him with the list of answers already prepared. Remember, in saving him time you are speeding up the time when he can bring you some measure of relief.

What Can the Doctor Do for You?

Now let us suppose that you have a headache that persists and gets worse. Do yourself a favor by not trying to treat yourself. Go immediately to your family physician and insist on an evaluation by a neurologic specialist. The specialist will give you a battery of tests that should consist of the following:

• A complete neurologic examination, which checks your brain and other parts of your nervous system;

• A complete X-ray examination of your skull and cervical spine; that is, in the region of the neck. Cervical arthritic changes, possibly caused by a whiplash injury, can trigger headaches that persist;

• A radioisotope (atomic particle) brain scan. This test has simplified the study of patients with suspicious intracranial problems. It is safe, and one can undergo this test as an out-patient.

This examination or examinations will be the basis for your treatment. By this time you should be reassured that something can be done for your pain, for, as I pointed out above, only about 3 to 5 percent of all headaches fall into the extreme serious class.

Some Methods to Control or Treat Headaches

Headache is one of the most common symptoms that brings patients to doctors. Only nervousness, fatigue, and constipation come close to it as a source of human complaint. Most doctors who see patients with headaches have come to accept the reality that their patients have already tried to treat themselves with every known drug on the market. The patient is now ready for help and wants no fooling around.

So to avoid fooling around, a good physician will evaluate his headache patient psychologically. Many times a person's headache is caused by something that is bothering him in his life-style. I recall one patient who was suffering from nervousness but hesitated to see a doctor about that. She worried so much about her condition that she developed severe headaches. This is not an unusual case. People often develop the most severe headaches from suppressed desires, frustrations, social setbacks, financial troubles, and just plain boredom. Some develop headaches because they subconsciously want somebody to help them.

A Routine for Treating Headaches

After many years of treating headache patients, I have arrived at the following routines for my own practice:

After a complete examination I decide if the patient is a good candidate for drug therapy. If I decide that drugs will help the patient, I insist that they be used on a regularly fixed schedule. This means that I insist that my patients take a certain dose at a certain time. I do not want them gulping down the medication just because their headache suddenly comes back. They must wait for the regular medication schedule.

Do I get arguments about this? You can bet your life! One indignant lady said very pointedly that she came to a doctor to get something to take when she hurt and not to take whenever he felt like giving the medicine to her. But let me add hastily that this routine is not arbitrary. It has a very sound basis. It fits into concepts of modern psychology known as operant conditioning. It is a method used to break the habit of rushing to the medicine cabinet each time you get a headache. Instead, you recondition yourself to tolerate headache pain for a certain interval and only to take drugs at a fixed time. You'll soon learn that you don't need as many drugs as you thought you did.

I then work out a schedule of physical measures for my headache patient. There is a simple relaxing technique I like to show them. You just relax on a sofa or a table and let your head hang over the edge to relax your tight neck muscles. Remember that it is spasms in these muscles that cause a lot of headaches.

Also, I recommend using a hand massager to vibrate the back of your neck. And sometimes when you come home with a headache, the application of a hot pack around the neck helps greatly. Followed by a massage, it is enough to relax you and break up those muscle spasms.

And lastly, if you feel a headache at night, try taking two aspirin, a warm bath, and some warm milk. It also helps if you forego jive, rock 'n' roll, and the "Anvil Chorus" on your stereo. Settle this time for some soft music. You may have forgotten how soothing it can be.

Special Techniques for Headache Relief

If the basic routines described above fail to bring relief, then we consider some special techniques. Among these are:

CERVICAL TRACTION

A home traction setup, which you can buy, is worth applying to further relax your neck muscles. Five to ten minutes of using five- to ten-pound weights is usually sufficient to relax your neck muscles to the point where your headache spasm will break up.

At the same time apply a hot pack around your neck. This can be made up of a Turkish towel folded and soaked in hot water and then wrung out carefully. Be careful you don't burn yourself while doing this.

INJECTION

I have mentioned before the value of Novocain injections into muscles as a pain relief measure. Such injections into tight neck muscles in the back of the head have worked when other methods have failed to relax them. Such injections cannot be given by yourself, of course. They are of limited value, but in the right circumstances they can be a great help when given by an expert.

ACUPUNCTURE

The value of acupuncture as a headache relief has come up many times since this ancient Chinese art became fashionable in the West. The Chinese claim good results in using it for headaches. I am personally satisfied that about one out of four headache sufferers can be helped—if they are willing to submit to three or four acupuncture treatments. However, acupuncture is still too recent—too recent to us, that is—for us to clearly evaluate its possibilities in this type of relief.

SURGICAL TECHNIQUES

There is limited value in neurosurgery as a relief of headaches that will not respond to more ordinary treatments. Recently Dr. Norman Shealy, a neurosurgeon, reported relief of certain types of headaches by a surgical interruption of fine nerves that come out of the cervical (neck) spine. He does this under X-ray control with a radiofrequency type of electrical current. This technique, while interesting, is too recent to evaluate.

Other methods of cutting nerves in the back of the head have sometimes added more misery to the chronic headache sufferer than the operation is worth. I have seen many patients operated on in this manner who have had more trouble after the surgery because of the numb sensation or the burning in the area caused by the lack of nerves.

This does not condemn all surgical treatment. Its use depends upon the specific cause of the headache. An occasional patient may have a localized pain over the back of the head. This may be due to injury to the occipital nerve or entrapment of the greater occipital nerve that supplies this area. The occipital area is that portion of the head occupied by the occipital bone, which forms the back part of the skull. A small percentage of patients can be helped by a simple operation of cutting this nerve.

Psychotherapy for Treatment of Headaches

The majority of headaches are associated with emotional tension. If this has been demonstrated, then why can't more patients be helped by psychotherapy?

Perhaps the reason is that the patient with headaches does not consider himself emotionally disturbed to the point where he needs to spend hours with a psychiatrist or clinical psychologist. So the percentage of patients who will submit to this method of treatment is small.

Those who have consulted psychotherapists have learned that their headaches were a part of a deeper emotional problem. Pain, as I have tried to point out many times in this book, has different levels of meaning.

First, the pain is a signal that something unpleasant is going on inside the body. If it is a specific pain whose source can be pinpointed, as with a toothache, the problem is simple. But when the pain is persistent and its cause indeterminate, then the pain reaches a different level of meaning in our minds. For some of us the level of meaning may be an expression of resentment, an attitude of anger, or a release of hostility. We may not even be aware of this association until it is pointed out to us through a psychologist's or psychiatrist's help.

It is still a mystery how a headache can be triggered by anger, resentment, hostility, or frustration in not getting what we want out of life. In the same manner, we have no real explanation at this time as to why the same emotional symptoms that cause an ulcer in one businessman will cause a chronic headache in another or cause a third person to develop high blood pressure. Theoretically, one would suppose that the same emotional symptoms would trigger the same physical reactions, but they certainly don't do so. There are theories as to why this difference in reaction occurs, but none of the theories have enough facts to support them.

The methods of psychotherapy generally allow the patient to ventilate or get rid of things that are bothering him. By telling the psychotherapist what is "eating him," the patient may get much relief from his chronic headache.

All of us have heard "body language" used to describe various aches and pains. For example, you may have had a disagreeable time with your boss and afterward used an expression, "He gives me a headache." In many cases this may be more than just an expression or play on words. He—or others ranging from friends, spouses, public officials, to clerks in stores—may be literally making your head ache.

Some Points to Remember about Headaches

Some basic points about headaches were brought out in the above discussion. These will help you understand the basic nature of your trouble. They are:

• Chronic headache is most often associated with emotional tension.

• If you have never suffered from headaches before, then by all means see your doctor at once. You need a thorough checkup, for common emotional tension is less likely to be causing your discomfort.

• If you have suffered from headaches for years and the *character* of your headaches changes, as in Larry's case, see a doctor at once. A new complication may have entered your case.

• Sinus trouble, eye trouble, high blood pressure, and other less common causes are not as important as emotional tension in generating headaches.

• If you are overdosing yourself with aspirin or similar widely advertised compounds, then see your doctor and have a complete evaluation.

• The medical profession is more aware of headaches today than ever before. Many specialists are interested in finding the causes. But you must be willing to accept the fact that your headache may be associated with emotional tension. This is extremely difficult for some patients to face. But the first step in treating emotional tension headaches must come from the patient. He must take steps to help himself. These steps include submitting to a thorough examination and—perhaps—undergoing psychotherapy to get to the bottom of the cause of the pain.

• Self-relief of headaches, once you know the cause, consists of following a routine of regular drug treatments, massage with a vibrator, and home cervical traction.

8

BACKACHES AND SCIATICA

No one knows for sure the true number of Americans who suffer from chronic backache. The National Center of Health statistics recently indicated that 6.3 million people in the United States suffer from back problems. Then, a recent issue of a national magazine claimed the figure was really closer to eight million.

That is a lot of pain, regardless of which set of figures you accept. You may wonder why the back is such a problem. It is because the back is the pole on which our bodies are hung. Subconsciously we acknowledge the back's importance in many of our everyday expressions. We say, "He has a lot of backbone," to indicate a person of strong character. Likewise, we call an indecisive person "spineless." All this indicates that we realize that man is characterized by his ability to stand straight because of his backbone.

Man is unique in this respect. If you will look at the animals in a zoo, you will see no other animal who stands bolt upright as man does. Monkeys, apes, and gorillas may stand on two legs, but they lack man's straightness. Whether this is a mark of human superiority or not is an open question, for man's upright position is the source of his chronic back problems.

Recent studies in the field have confirmed that the sedentary way of life we lead today and our push-button culture may account for an excessive increase of back problems in the last twenty-five years.

The Back as a Target of Emotional Disturbance

Hans Kraus, of New York University Medical Center, is one of the outstanding experts on nonsurgical treatments of chronic back problems. He has done numerous studies to indicate that faulty muscle function in the low back and abdominal muscles account for much of our chronic back trouble. He quotes one study made using a technique called electromyography, which makes electric measurements of the back muscles. It showed that during anxiety-provoking interviews patients under study had an excessive electrical discharge from the muscles of the spine.

Kraus has also been a proponent of the "trigger point" theory by demonstrating that under the skin and in the areas of certain muscles there are tiny zones of fibrosis. This is a hardening of the tissues surrounding the muscles. He believes that the painful points arise from these hardened tissue zones. Kraus has demonstrated his belief by injecting small amounts of Novocain into the areas of these painful trigger points. He succeeded in relieving some severe back pains.

The back has also become a psychosomatic target organ. One of the most common causes of psychosomatically triggered physical disorders is the constantly upset stomach suffered by the person who works under tension. A diagnosis of stomach ulcer is a frequent finding in such cases. High blood pressure, asthma, certain forms of arthritis, some chronic headaches, and various other pains are all part of the psychosomatic galaxy.

A considerable amount of back pain may quite possibly be

in the same class. However, proof of a psychosomatic cause for backache is not as simple as the electromyographic recordings of excessive muscle potentials. Kraus conducted during anxiety-provoking interviews might suggest. Much more study needs to be done on this.

Why We Have Back Pains

The best way to understand why mankind suffers chronic back problems is to examine the structure of the spine. The trouble lies in the inherent nature of the spinal column. It is true that lack of exercise does not help maintain strong back muscle tone, but many athletes who are constantly working their muscles are victims of back problems. However, there is certainly a greater incidence of backache among sedentary workers. Kraus did a study on psychoanalysts who spend most of their time sitting down listening to patients. The incidence of chronic backache in this professional group was exceedingly high.

It would appear that people who have to stand would put a much greater strain on their spines than people who do their work sitting down. Therefore, they should have a greater incidence of back trouble. This might be true if everyone sat correctly, but a slouching posture while sitting may put more strain on the spine than standing correctly.

Basic Structure of the Spine

The spine is made up of a series of bones called vertebras, which are connected. The word *vertebra* means "twisted." It received this name because the components that make up the basic units of the spine have a twisted look. The vertebra consists of a block of bone that is basically kidney-shaped. An arch of bone is attached to this, making up the vertebral canal.

A vertebra is not the functional unit of the spine, however. The functional unit consists of two vertebras joined by a disc. The disc looks simple, but in reality it is extremely complex. Also, it is poorly understood. You can think of the disc as a tough band of rubbery tissue that is wrapped around a fluid center. Even this is not entirely accurate, because the fluid (*nucleus pulposus*) is really a gel.

You can compare the disc to the shock absorber on a car or you can compare it to a washer that is placed between two metal parts to absorb vibration. The disc differs from a washer in that it is a living structure. Its main duty is to permit us to bend our spines in various directions. If there were no discs between the vertebral bones, man's spine would be stiff. He would be unable to move his spine.

This rigidity of the spine is what tragically happens in cases of advanced arthritis. The disc is absorbed by the body and replaced by calcium, causing the individual vertebras to fuse together in one continuous bone.

The disc makes up a significant part of the human spine. The fluid or gel that it contains is a living chemical substance made up of polysaccharides and protein. Since it is a living structure, the fluid in the disc itself can increase or decrease in tiny amounts. You can test this for yourself by noting that a person's height can be less in the evening than it is in the morning. Measure you height very precisely the first thing in the morning and again in the evening. You may be amazed to see that there is definitely a small difference.

Some anatomists believe that this is due to the fluid content of the disc being less in the evening. Then, during sleep and rest the fluid finds its way back into the disc. As we grow older we become shorter in stature, because the disc loses its natural water content and strength. This can cause us to lose inches from our height as we get older.

These vertebral bodies and the discs make up the functional units of the spine. Around these structures are the numerous muscles that move the spine. The muscles of the back and the abdomen are of great importance, since they maintain posture and permit us to move our spines.

You can experiment with yourself in this regard. Lie on your back and just raise your neck. Now try to roll your knees upward toward your chest. As you do, place your hands on your abdominal muscles, and you will feel them harden. The movement of bending your body forward is done by the abdominal muscles and the deep muscles of the spine.

In contrast, when you bend to the right, to the left, or backwards, you bend with the muscles that form the tough columns on either side of the spine. The spine in its entirety runs from the base of the skull down to the tail bone. The natural curve in the lower back is a gentle one and is concave in its low back portion.

The spine is called the *vertebral column.* The vertebral arch portion of the spine is extremely important because it protects the cablelike structure of the spinal cord that connects the brain with the muscles and skin.

The number of movements performed every minute by the human back is hard to imagine. When you stand erect, the muscles of the spine are in constant rhythmical contraction. This is just like those of the knee. Without this contraction you would fall to the ground. Even when you sit down, the spinal muscles are constantly adjusting themselves.

Now let's consider the nerves that come out of the vertebral or spinal canal. Two bones, you will remember, make up a spinal functional unit. These vertebras have notches in them. The top one, in the functional unit of two, has a concave notch that curves downward. The lower bone has a concave notch that curves upward. The two notches together form a canal known as a *foramen.* This foramen or hole in the vertebral canal is the exit point of the spinal nerve. This nerve leaves the spinal canal and breaks up into feeling or sensory portions and into a motor portion to move muscles. All the feeling that goes from the skin backward to the spinal canal must pass through the boney canal or boney-notched foramen. The front of that notch (foramen) is bordered by the disc and the back portion of the ligaments and bones. The joint that connects the two vertebral portions of the arch is known as a *facet.*

This arrangement of bones, disc, muscles, and nerves offers an endless number of possibilities for backaches. The vertebral bones themselves are painless. The disc or shock absorber between the vertebral bodies, which help give movement to the spine, is also painless. The tough fibrous tissue (*annulus fibrosus*) that holds the disc in place has some tiny nerves that are supplied by the spinal nerve. The joint in the lower spine (facet), which allows for the gliding movement of bending forward and backward, is a true joint. Consequently, it can be attacked by all kinds of arthritis problems.

The spinal nerve that goes through the foramen can also be a source of painful conditions; for example, neuritis.

Some Common Causes of Backache and Sciatica

Considering the complex arrangement of the spinal column and the way it works, it does not take much imagination to visualize the many conditions that can cause a backache and irritation of a nerve root. A common condition is when the pain shoots into the leg. This is called sciatica, after the sciatic nerve, which is affected in this painful condition.

Backache can come from multiple causes. One authority

lists over a hundred distinct causes. A practical approach, however, is for the practicing physician to group those causes that can be extremely serious or dangerous for his patient. Then he groups those that are important, but not of dangerous significance.

The percentage of serious backache cases is about the same as that of serious headache cases. At least 90 percent or more of ordinary headaches are associated with emotional tension. Another 5 percent is attributed to migraine. Thus, 95 percent of common headaches are not of a serious or dangerous significance. Only 5 percent indicate a potentially dangerous condition in the patient.

So it is with backaches. It is now believed that 90 percent or more of backaches are due to faulty posture and a chronic muscle flabbiness. In other words, if you have a backache, the chances are 90 percent or more that your problem is due to faulty posture, lack of muscle tone, or hyperkinetic (abnormal muscular movement) disorder and not to a serious condition.

I also feel that we can place in the 90 percent nonserious class arthritic problems of the spine, which I feel have been exaggerated. In the same class is the so-called degenerative disease of the discs, which I discussed earlier. This diagnosis has filled too many patients with unnecessary fear. It happens to all of us over forty.

When I speak of 90 percent of backaches as being of a nonserious nature, I do not wish to imply that they don't hurt. They often do and definitely need treatment. They can be helped. Generally this help is special exercises to strengthen the muscles and to correct posture. In extreme cases muscular injections of Novocain may be indicated.

The important point is that the majority of backaches are not serious and can be taken care of. But then what about the other 10 percent that are serious complications?

The So-called Slipped Disc Syndrome

Up to now I have not mentioned the slipped disc syndrome except in brief reference in a few case histories where a ruptured disc pressed on the spinal nerve. It is certainly a very painful disorder, but again I feel that this diagnosis has been overworked tremendously.

First, let me say that the term *slipped disc* is a bad one, although not as frightening as *degenerative arthritis*. In reality there is no such thing as slippage of a disc. This "shock absorber" between the vertebral bodies is poorly named. It is not flat and lifeless. As I explained earlier in the description of the spine, the disc is a living structure. It is shaped like a flattened egg and is still elliptical. It constantly changes its fluid content, and its chemical content is subject to many biological alterations.

The term *slipped disc* sounds like the material between the vertebras is a flat, disclike object that jumps out of place when we make faulty movements or our backs "lock." This is far from the case and the reason why the concept that the back can be manipulated into a correct position has not been proved. Chiropractic manipulation and osteopathic adjustment of the spine have their places. They can in some cases relieve an acute backache. But they do not achieve this relief by mechanically pushing a slipped disc back into place between the vertebras.

Ask any chiropractor or osteopathic surgeon, and he will gladly tell you that he is snapping the facets that join the spine together much like you pull your knuckles and hear a cracking. Then what does happen when we have a condition called a slipped disc? The back has an inherent structural weakness. As time passes, the tough ligament or muscle that holds the disc in place thins out considerably. Then, an unusual stress, twist, turn, or bending to lift an excessive weight can cause the vertebral bones to squeeze the disc material between them, causing the disc to push or bulge backward into the vertebral canal.

As I described earlier, the front portion of the foramen, (hole) through which the nerve root passes, is bordered by the side of the disc itself. It is possible for the disc to rupture or herniate—that is, to be pushed out of its regular place—and to compress this nerve root.

This is a common occurrence and happens more often than we appreciate. When the disc ruptures, it causes pain by compressing the nerve that goes to the spinal root nerve. This causes muscles along the spine to go into a spasm to protect the body from further harm. Often this muscular spasm will tilt a person's body away from the side of the rupture.

If the disc material (*nucleus pulposus*) has ruptured completely, then a mechanical situation is set up where a piece of the disc jams into the foramen. This causes a chronic irritation of the nerve root. When this happens, pain extends into the leg or along the sciatic nerve distribution. The sciatic nerve runs down the back of the thigh.

Fortunately, ruptured discs that generate sciatic nerve troubles are not common. Most of the early backache problems, I repeat, are due to muscle sprain or faulty use of the spine, either in poor posture or improper lifting of heavy objects. However, the 2 or 3 percent of back sufferers who do have ruptured discs face unpleasant consequences. These include weak structures, weak tissues, and a possible pain in the leg or into the back. This can be extremely disabling. disabling.

Cases of Typical Low Back Problems

All this discussion of the anatomy and mechanics of the lower back and spine was to provide background so you could understand various case reports that illustrate the commonest causes of backache and what we can do to help you when it happens to your own back.

The first case is Bill and his flabby back muscles. Bill is a thirty-three-year-old insurance executive. When he first developed a nagging backache, Bill sought the best medical advice he knew: a friend who had once had a backache himself. He had always believed that "experience is the best teacher," as he was fond of pointing out. The advice wasn't free by any means. Bill had to buy the drinks as they discussed his problem at a bar one day.

The friend knew exactly what was wrong. The same thing had happened to him. It was all due to a poor chair that was putting a strain on his back. This sounded reasonable, and cheered by the experienced advice, Bill bought himself a new chair for his office. The back was straight as he had been advised to buy, but it didn't seem to help at all.

Next he decided, "Well, it will go away." But it didn't. So he finally got around to seeing his doctor. He spent several hundred dollars for X rays of his lower spine and for blood and other necessary tests. Still his condition did not improve. Too impatient to realize that it takes time to run down causes of deep-seated troubles, he quit his doctor in disgust.

He next turned to a back specialist that a friend had recommended. The new doctor told him frankly that his trouble did not come from excessive and improper sitting as Bill had originally thought. It was due, the doctor told him, to loss of tone in the muscles of his lower back.

Bill couldn't have disagreed more. He pointed out somewhat acidly that when he was in the Marines he could make a ten-mile hike "without raising a sweat."

"When did you leave the Corps?" the doctor asked mildly.

It had been nine years ago, when Bill was twenty-four. He took his discharge, married, and joined his father's insurance agency.

"Let's try a little test," the doctor said. He had Bill lie down on an examination table. He held his patient's knees to keep them from buckling and asked Bill to sit up. The best Bill could do, lying on his back, was to barely raise his shoulders off the table.

"What did you weigh when you got out of the Corps?" the doctor asked, motioning for Bill to get on the scales. "One sixty-five," Bill replied. "But I've probably picked up a few pounds since then."

The needle of the scales shot up to 215 pounds. Questioned about what sports he participated in, Bill admitted that he had taken up golf but soon dropped it. His recreation consisted almost entirely of watching football on TV, driving fast boats and big cars, and drinking beer.

Deflated by his poor physical showing, Bill now kept quiet and listened for a change. He was told that he had practically no performance in his abdominal muscles and only a minimal amount in his low back muscles.

"These muscles are what holds up your spine," Bill was told. "Unfortunately, you've neglected them and now you're paying for it."

"I just don't understand," Bill said, shaking his head with a worried look on his face. "I was always tough as a boot."

"Surprisingly enough," the doctor replied, "former athletes sometimes have more back trouble than less active men."

"I suppose that's because their backs and spines take a beating on the gridiron," Bill said.

"It might seem so, but competing athletes are in good shape. Their muscles have good tone and are strong enough to protect them. Their trouble starts only when they stop playing and put on weight—like somebody I *just* happen to know."

Bill grinned weakly and then grimaced as a sudden spasm of pain hit his back. "Okay," he said. "I'm sold. What do I do now, coach?"

The back specialist put Bill on the following routine:

• *Severe weight reduction.* He was given a diet to follow that eliminated all starches and substituted a glass of milk for each six-pack of beer he formerly consumed.

• *Muscle toning program.* This consisted of eight basic exercises which I will discuss later. This physical improvement program was supervised by the specialist and the therapist in his office.

• *Proper rest.* This included throwing away his soft mattress and getting one firm enough to support his sagging back.

• *Daily isometric exercises.* These exercises, which he could do while sitting in his office, supplemented the supervised muscle-toning program devised by his doctor.

• *A walking program.* He was ordered to avoid elevators and to climb stairs. He found a parking place a half-mile from his office and added a mile's walk each day to his regular routine.

The change in his sedentary way of life was hard to take at first, but with his back pain to nag him on, Bill stuck to it. As his sagging muscles began to tighten up, his backache gradually improved. Today, he still follows a common sense approach to his body and is seldom bothered by his old back trouble. All his previous pain had been due to the inability of his flabby muscles to properly support his spinal column.

The Exercise Addict

Bill's case would seem to indicate that exercise is the specific remedy for a large number of back troubles. This is quite true. Exercise is the key to treatment in many back trouble cases. But on the other hand, what about Arthur? He was an exercise nut and he had back trouble too.

Arthur was a fifty-four-year-old lawyer. He had been

turned down for insurance when he was thirty-six because of overweight and high blood pressure. The refusal frightened him, and he turned into an exercise addict. Arthur's father had died prematurely of a heart attack. Arthur had been warned that unless he brought his weight down and toned up his body, he was also a candidate for the same tragic end.

This was good advice, but unfortunately, Arthur was a man who believed wholeheartedly in self-determination. The rule of his life was, "If you want something, go after it!" He was a hard-driving, self-made man who had never stopped working since he was twelve years old. So when he was told by his doctor that he needed exercise and dieting, Arthur went at both with the same do-or-die spirit that had carried him to the top of the legal profession. He literally became an exercise nut. He tried all the standard ones and then added every fad from isometrics to the Royal Canadian Air Force Fitness Program.

Then he discovered tennis and handball. He lived in Philadelphia and in the winter months played handball at the end of each day and on weekends. In the warmer months he used outdoor courts and played hard-driving tennis.

At fifty-two he was in relatively good shape and suddenly decided to add skiing to his list of sports. Unable to do anything moderately, he wanted to skip the "snow bunny" class and go directly into cross-country skiing and high jumping. Arthur's physician warned him against this, but he paid no attention. Then after several spills due to faulty landings on his jumps, Arthur developed a chronic backache. His idea of treatment was to "work the kinks out."

One day he gave his low back region more punishment than it could take. He was attempting a cross-country run when he turned over in a deep, unexpected snowbank. He thought at first that he had broken his leg, for he felt savage shooting pains in his left leg extending from his hip to his big toe. He lay in the snow, bent over like a pretzel. He was unable to get up, and a rescue party had to carry him on a stretcher to a nearby hospital.

Arthur's back was locked in a spasm. He could move his leg and toes on command, but any excessive elevation of his left leg was unbearable. His only position of comfort was on his side with both of his knees drawn up toward his chest. He was transferred by special ambulance to a Philadelphia hospital. There he spent fourteen days lying on his back with his legs and hips pulled by twenty-pound traction weights. Those two weeks were plain torture for him. His doctors tried to stand him up, but the pain was unbearable. They had to give him regular injections of narcotics to relieve his agony.

Various specialists and consultants were called in to see him. Novocain was injected into the muscles in his lower back. This relieved some of the spasm of Arthur's lower back but did not help the sciatic pain at all.

X rays of his lower back showed that the discs had been badly worn at the third, fourth, and fifth lumbar (near the loins) spaces. A neurologic specialist then found that Arthur's left ankle jerk was absent and that there was persistent pain on raising the patient's left leg. It was his opinion that there was pressure on Arthur's sciatic nerve but felt that it might respond to conservative treatment. He advised another week in traction, coupled with daily physical therapy.

Arthur submitted to this routine and recovered from the worst of his pain. He left the hospital wearing a heavy low-back corset. He was warned not to participate in any strenuous sports, especially skiing. But after sixteen years of depending upon exercise as the solution to all his bodily ills, he could not break his old habits. He began with a program of routine swimming, which was one of the best things he could do. His residual pain gradually diminished. Then he resumed his old strenuous sports of handball and running. During one handball game he twisted his back and brought on a second attack of severe pain in his hip and left leg. He was taken back to the hospital, but this time bed rest and traction of his pelvis were not sufficient to relieve his excruciating pain.

He was told that his previous skiing accident had most probably ruptured a fragment of disc material in his low back area. The pressure this had placed on his spinal nerve had been relieved by bed rest and traction, but this new injury had now aggravated the original rupture. His doctors recommended a myelogram test to verify the diagnosis.

After numbing the lumbar (near the loins) area of his spine, dye was injected into the subarachnoid space of his lower spine. The resulting X rays, with the contrast made possible by the dye's reaction to the radiation, disclosed a defect at the fifth lumbar vertebra level (L5). A piece of his ruptured disc was pressing on the spinal nerve.

This was basically the same thing he had experienced before. So he felt encouraged and envisioned a couple of weeks in traction and then recovery. He was told that his condition was much worse than it had been before. There was a possibility that his injury could respond to conservative treatment but would take far more time than it had before—if it worked at all. In the meantime he would have to endure his pain. If he found this unacceptable, he was told, surgical treatment would bring more rapid relief.

The neurosurgeon explained to Arthur that surgical treatment would *not* give him "a new back." His trouble was caused by abuse of his back and spine through too active exercise at an age when he should have been slowing up. The need for an operation was not urgent, because there was no weakness yet in his legs. However, his pain was unbearable. If he were placed on narcotics to relieve the pain while more conservative treatment was tried, there was a strong possibility of him becoming an addict. The drug doses would gradually lose their ability to deaden his excruciating pain and would have to be gradually increased to afford relief. With recovery expected to be slow, the need for narcotic relief would be prolonged past the point of safety.

Faced with these dreadful alternatives, Arthur readily agreed to a laminectomy, as this particular spinal operation is called. The surgeon subsequently removed a large fragment of the *nucleus pulposus* that had ruptured out of the intervertebral disc. The nerve root had been jammed in the foramen. This jamming was why Arthur failed to obtain relief from the usual measures of rest.

He made a rapid recovery after his operation, but within a month of his operation he foolishly returned to active exercise. The last I heard of him he was again suffering from chronic back pain and recurrent sciatica.

Comments

Excessive exercise ruined Arthur's back. This is not to say that he should have lapsed into a sedentary life. Then he would have opened himself to the same type of trouble as Bill, in our previous case history. But Arthur should have settled for a calmer type of exercise. He was definitely on the right road with his swimming routines. Swimming not only exercises all our muscles, but the gentle pressure of the water helps support our muscles, and the water's movement is a mild form of water therapy. Older readers may recall that swimming was the major exercise prescribed for President Franklin D. Roosevelt who had lost the use of his legs due to polio. A heated pool was built in the White House basement especially for his use. Another was built at his retreat in Warm Springs, Georgia.

Arthur might also have added a few light rounds of golf to

his routine. If he had restricted his activity to exercises that would have maintained muscle tone without putting stress and strain on his weakened spine, it is unlikely that he would have suffered additional pain. His was a case of poor tissue that was abused. His case represents about 2 percent of those who suffer from backache and sciatica.

Nancy and Her Fusion

Nancy had always been active and never suffered from backache until she married and became pregnant for the third time in six years. Then in the third month of her pregnancy, with two highly active children to see after, she started complaining of daily nagging pains in her lower back. In the early morning she was just as full of zip and freedom from pain as ever, but by the middle of the day her pains began. By nightfall the pain was almost unbearable. The pain was all concentrated in her back. It did not extend into her legs as pressure on the sciatic nerve does.

Her obstetrician told her that the frequency of her pregnancies may have caused overrelaxation of the structures of her lower spine. She then obtained some relief by taking a squatting position when lifting objects and using a hard mattress to support her spine at night. By the time she was in her ninth month of pregnancy, she was in constant pain and spent much of her time in bed. This put a heavy strain on her husband, Tom. After working all day, he had to come home to do the chores and watch after the children. They had no money to hire anyone to help out, and both their relatives lived too far away to be of any assistance. Life became very difficult for the entire family.

They both hoped that Nancy's condition would improve after her child was delivered. When it did not, she undertook a series of X rays. They disclosed that her lower spine had an abnormal position of the vertebra. Her condition is known as a "slippage" or medically as *spondylolisthesis.* In her case it was a birth defect in the structure of her spine that had showed itself under the stress of repeated childbearing.

Her condition was helped by rest but was brought back by any excessive lifting. With babies to bathe and diaper, meals to cook, and a house to care for, it was impossible for her to avoid all lifting. In desperation she consulted a bone specialist. He advised her that she had to accept the limitation of her weak spine or submit to a fusion operation. The fusion operation would remove the disc between the offending vertebras and fuse or grow them together.

Unable to face the thought of an operation, Nancy tried back-strengthening exercises, swimming, and wearing a firm back brace of steel supports. None of these brought her any significant relief. She then submitted to wearing a plaster cast for three months. For the first time she obtained complete relief from her nagging back pain, but the cast was a discomfort and an inconvenience.

At this point she finally gave in to the operation. After a successful fusion of her lower spine, Nancy was improved enough to carry on normal living with freedom from pain. Unfortunately, she had to avoid any more pregnancies. She and Tom took necessary measures to assure this.

Comments

I included this case history to show that in a very small percent of patients—perhaps less than 1 percent—there may be a true abnormal spine structure causing the back pain. Although this rarely occurs, it shows the importance of having a thorough examination of the lumbar spine and low back area by qualified specialists. I included this case for another reason as well. Earlier I discussed the large number of headaches and back pains that appear to have an emotional tension cause. This case points out that not every person with chronic backache is a psychoneurotic. Nancy was highly motivated and wanted children. Her painful condition was not a psychosomatic reaction to frequent pregnancies. She was unfortunately born with a weak spine.

What You Can Do If You Have Chronic Low Backaches

• *Study the pattern of the backache.* You must know the *when, where, why,* and *how* of your pain. The more intelligently you can answer these questions, the better you can help yourself when you do consult a physician.

• *Invest in a complete examination.* It can be done by your family doctor or by a specialist. Your condition, like Nancy's, may not be what it appears to be on the surface.

• *Learn the proper way to use your back.* This means squatting down instead of bending when you lift things. This places the strain on your legs instead of your back.

• *Don't be an athlete addict like our attorney friend.* Exercises are necessary to maintain muscle tone and insure that we do not get backaches from sagging muscles. But at the same time exercises must be adjusted to the individual body.

What To Do If You Are Suddenly Hit by Back Pain

Suppose you bend over to tie your shoe or stoop to pick up something and suddenly find that you can't straighten up again. Your back is locked in a painful spasm. The first rule is "Don't panic." When this happens, it is amazing the number of victims who imagine the worst will happen to them. What you should do is remind yourself that you most likely have a muscle spasm with a bruising of the muscle and that rest will help you.

If this happens, I advise you to do something like this:

• Try to lie on the floor and bring your knees up sharply to your chest. You can hope that this will break up the spasm and unlock your muscles.

• You may have to lie on the floor or ground for a few minutes with your knees up toward your chest. Take a deep breath and try to relax your muscles. Get someone to help you to a hard board or sofa.

Now you are taken home and still have a pain in your back. What do you do now? At this point I recommend plenty of heat. It can be in the form of a hot towel to make a moist hot pack or a commercial product you can buy called a Hydrocollater. If you can be put into a hot tub of water with Epsom salts (or even table salt), you will find that the muscle will relax.

Now you must get off your feet completely. Gravity, or the upright position, is the worst enemy you have when your back is in severe pain. The back pain is a signal that is trying to tell you to put your muscles and joints to rest for a while. So make up your mind that you are in for some days of bed rest. You will need a firm mattress or a plywood board (about an inch thick) between the springs and mattress.

You should also try to have everything at your bedside, so you will not have to get out of bed for anything except to go to the bathroom. A bedside commode, which you can rent, will be helpful, for it will save you the strain of going to the bathroom.

This routine may sound harsh, but there is no simple way to break up a muscle spasm without going into a hospital for bed rest. After several days of rest, forcing yourself to stay in bed, you should start feeling better. During this time you should drink plenty of fluids, but do not worry about eating regular meals. Incidentally, this is a good time and way to reduce.

Exercises for Bad Backs

There are two basic types of exercises. Isometric exercises are those in which there are no basic movements. Muscles are pitted against themselves or immovable objects. Isotonic exercises are those in which movement plays a part. Both types are used for strengthening the back. Here are some of them:

• A simple isometric exercise technique for strengthening the low back muscles is to stand with your back against a wall. Then, tighten your buttocks. By doing so you also tighten the muscles on either side of your spine.

• Now try this. Lie on your back and bring first one knee and then the other up to your chest. Tighten your buttocks as you alternately move your knees.

• Here is a gentle exercise to strengthen your abdominal muscles. Lie flat on your back, face up. Now gently lift your shoulders off the floor. Do not help with your hands. Let all the lift come from tightening your abdominal and back muscles. This need not be done vigorously. As you raise up, put your hands on your abdomen and feel the muscles tighten up. After you get some practice at this, you can raise your shoulders, count to ten, and then lower your shoulders slowly to the floor. This is a simple exercise, but it goes a long way toward putting tone back into your muscles.

• Now sit on the edge of a table and swing your hip backward and forward. This will help tighten the buttock muscles and also help the bender and flexor muscles of the hip.

• Deep knee bends are essential if you want to protect your back in the future. Stand straight and hold onto a chair for support as you squat down and then raise yourself up. This is the position you should take if you are going to pick up a heavy object. The lifting strain will then be placed on your legs and thighs instead of your bent back. Deep knee bends will strengthen your legs so they can easily take this strain.

Some other rules you should follow are:

• Avoid sleeping face down on your stomach. This is the worst possible position for your back. During the hours of sleep your muscles relax. Your back is bent backward if you sleep on your stomach. We call this hyperextended. As we age and the joints in our spine become thinner, compression of nerve roots can easily take place under this condition. This is why many "belly sleepers" awake with backaches. Never mind reminding me that babies sleep this way. Their backs are still elastic and they have plenty of free movement. You and I do not have it.

• Avoid vigorous sports like running, jogging, skiing, and hard tennis if you are not really keeping up muscle tone. These vigorous activities are not for the weekend sportsman unless you want to risk injury to your back. Swimming, on the other hand, is an excellent sport, as I pointed out earlier. It is recommended by all specialists who treat back problems.

Importance of Avoiding Nervous Tension

You must be tired by now of hearing doctors tell you to avoid nervous tension. Yet, whether we talk about headaches, sleeplessness, or backaches, we always come back to a warning about the dangers of nervous tension. This is not another slice of the same old baloney. There is sufficient documentation to prove that nervousness and tense muscles contribute to chronic headaches, irritable bowels, stomach disorders, insomnia, and backache as well.

The reason for this is that we move our bodies as a whole unit. One small action may put strain on other parts of the body. Stop and consider the effort put out in the simple task of opening a jar. It doesn't come easy. The lid is stuck. So what happens to our bodies? We tighten our fingers, the muscles of our arms, and our backs. But at the same time we tighten our jaws, grit our teeth, and grimace.

Now stop and think it over. What contribution to removing a tight lid does tightening the jaw muscles and gritting our teeth do? You really open the jar with your hands, you know. This shows that we are tensing and using unnecessary muscles. The next time you have to wait for someone or your boss gives you a job you dislike you'll find your body tensing and your jaw tightening. Here again we are using muscles and energy in wasted actions. Isn't it possible to resent the boss without putting a strain on our overworked bodies? We really need to use only a portion of the nervous energy we expend to get by in this modern world. The rest of it is just wasted. And as a result of this waste we develop nervous tension, making us the targets of psychosomatic headaches, low back pains, and other painful conditions.

I cannot tell you how to relax. This is something you must work out for yourself, for it directly involves your emotions. Nervous tension is probably the reason for both excessive smoking and excessive drinking. The victim is seeking help in trying to relax from the nervous tensions of everyday life.

Some Final Points

There are some final points concerning backache that I would like to leave with you. Some are new. Others I have mentioned before but are worth repeating.

• Try to stay calm by having a positive attitude toward life. Not everything that happens is a calamity. Most of us exaggerate our troubles and expect the worst.

• Your back was made to last a long time and will do so if

the muscles are kept strong. They are kept strong by proper exercises, and not violent exertions.

• Sit in hard-back chairs; sit tall, and stand tall, and avoid slouching.

• Your abdominal muscles play a strong part in maintaining a strong back, which surprises many people. Overeating and excessive weight weaken the abdominal muscles with a corresponding effect upon your back. I know this sounds like the stock cliche you get from every doctor at every visit: "Lose weight, cut out smoking." I wish I could tell you not to lose weight, but this would not be good advice. Excessive weight harms the back as well as other parts of the body. Keep tightening your diaphragm and belly muscles. Sometimes, for men, an abdominal support is a good idea.

• Try swimming a lot to maintain your back muscles.

• Remember that vigorous exercise, especially heavy contact sports such as touch football, basketball, and handball are all hazards for your low back region. Skiing, including water skiing, is a risky business for those of us who do not do it regularly.

• If you are stricken by severe backache, don't panic. It generally means muscle spasm or tearing of a low back muscle, which does not require any prolonged care or surgical treatment.

• Operations on the lower spine can be a blessing to those suffering the chronic pain of sciatica or pain down the leg. Fortunately these represent only a small percent of cases. But for those who fail to get help from bed rest, exercises, traction, heat, or injections into the muscles, surgery may provide welcome relief from chronic pain.

• Acupuncture has helped many patients who have chronic low back pain, but this method must not be tried without a thorough examination by competent physicians and specialists. Then perhaps one case out of four may be helped.

• Remember no one can give you a new back. No operation has yet been designed to replace the bad structures in the spine. Our discs, with care, should last a lifetime, but we do not have replacement parts if they don't. An operation will not give you a new spine, but it can relieve pain or a neurologic deficit like leg weakness.

• Lastly, do not consent to any operations on your lower back without the advice of several specialists. The only basis for surgery is to relieve pain. Many times this can be put off while you get opinions from several specialists.

9

WHIPLASH INJURIES: NECK AND ARM PAINS

The term *whiplash* was popularized some years ago by a neurosurgeon, and it refers to a sudden whiplike movement of the neck. Whiplash often occurs in a collision between two automobiles; the driver's head is thrown forward by the impact and then snaps backward. The stress and strain put on the vertebras at the neck is devastating.

A friend and patient of mine named Bert was waiting for a red light to change at an intersection when his car was struck hard in the rear by another vehicle. His head was thrown forward, his chin almost struck the steering wheel, and then his head snapped back. Instantly, he was struck with severe pain in the back of the neck where the upper part of the spinal column joins with the thorax.

Later, Bert described his sensations at the moment of impact. "I thought that seeing stars when you are struck was something that comic-strip artists had invented," he said. "But it happened. I saw stars, and they were all exploding. I thought the top of my head was going to blow off." He was also conscious of a strong tingling sensation in his hands. He had a horrified feeling that his neck was broken.

Bert was rushed to the hospital in an ambulance. In an unconscious effort to ease the pain in his neck, Bert held his hands behind his neck. It was the best thing he could have done, for it gave support to his badly strained vertebras. At the hospital the pain in the back of his neck increased. It throbbed, and an electric needle sensation radiated into his arms. He was more than ever certain that he had broken his neck. He began to panic, visualizing himself paralyzed for life.

The hospital doctors reassured him. They found no evidence of a fracture and advised that he had a severe muscle sprain in the neck. They placed a soft cervical collar made of felt around his neck and sent him home.

That night Bert felt worse. Pain increased in his neck. His head ached intensely, and he was in total discomfort. He tried to phone me, but I was out of town. The following day I saw him in my office. He came in guarding his neck as if it were broken. His face was drawn. His expression was anxious, and his body was tense. He gave me a vivid description of the accident and told me he thought he was going to die. Bert's personality is a highly emotional one, so I wasn't surprised at his reaction. He kept saying over and over, "You know, I could have been killed!"

My neurological examination showed that he was highly tensed. The muscles in the back of his neck were stiffened and very tender. He could barely move his neck and would not let me move it from side to side. However, his hand grips were good and strong, indicating that there had been no damage to his spinal cord. He had excellent movements in his arms, and his reflexes, when tested with a rubber hammer, were normal. He felt pin pricks, proving that sensation had not been disturbed. All of these tests told me that Bert's nervous system—that is, the spinal cord and nerves in his arms—had not been damaged by his injury.

I did my best to reassure Bert that he would survive his accident without any permanent injury, but ten days later I had to admit him to a hospital. What he needed most was complete rest to let his strained muscles recover, and he just wasn't getting it at home.

In the hospital he was forced to take complete bed rest in addition to traction and physical treatments to his neck. His traction was done with a special canvas halter that was placed around his chin and the back of his neck. The halter was connected to ten- to fifteen-pound weights by a rope that ran through a pulley, creating a constant pull on Bert's neck muscles. He also received hot packs on the back of his neck for about two weeks. Bert finally began to feel better.

Nevertheless, six months after the injury Bert was still complaining about pain in the back of the neck and was fearful of driving his car. Even when he rode as a passenger with me, Bert was apprehensive each time we stopped for a light. He insisted on wearing his cervical collar in the car and kept looking back, fearful that we would be struck by a car in our rear.

Bert's case is rather an extreme one due to his emotional reaction to the accident. In the most common type of whiplash injury the patient complains of pain in the back of his neck immediately after the accident. This generally becomes worse the next day but finally subsides after three or four weeks.

The Mechanisms Behind a Whiplash Injury

The cervical spine (the neck portion) is made up of seven bones that are connected to one another with ligaments. The spinal cord (of nerves) traverses the canal in the back of these bones. Between each set of bones there are discs and openings known as foramina (holes) and a nerve root that goes through them to supply impulses to the upper neck, back of the head, and the major nerves that innervate the arms. The cervical spine is subjected to a tremendous amount of movement, if you stop to think about it, in the course of a lifetime. If you add up all the times that you turn your head, nod, jerk, shake, and bend, it will add up to millions of movements. These millions of movements are wear and tear that produce changes in the joints of the spine.

The human spine is not built to withstand excessive injuries, just as the shock absorbers on your car will not stand up to excessive hard bumps in the road. When the cervical spine is snapped suddenly forward and then backward in a forceful, abrupt manner, there is a tearing of the ligaments that hold the vertebras. A cervical sprain occurs when this takes place. The muscles in the neck then go into spasm to protect the nerves from irritation. The trachea (windpipe) and the major blood vessels in the front of the neck that go to the brain may also be affected if the whiplash is serious enough.

Because of the number of structures that can be harmed when the head is thrown forward and then backward so abruptly, you may feel many different symptoms. These include:

• *Dizziness.* This may come from possible injury to nerves that go to the back of the head. It can also be due to irritation of blood vessels to the brain.

• *Tingling in the arms.* This condition arises from irritation of the nerve roots in the arms.

• *Watering of the eyes.* This is stimulated by the sympathetic nerves that go to the tear glands.

• *Severe headache.* This is caused by tearing of muscles in the back of the head and irritation of two large nerves that find their way there.

How Doctors Treat Whiplash Injuries

Bert's case history shows the general plan of treatment for a severe case of whiplash injury. It surprises a lot of people to learn that the best rule from the time of the first emergency treatment is best applied in moderation. By that I mean that there should be no more movement of the patient's neck than absolutely necessary, including the taking of many X rays.

The reason for this is that the slightest movement results in excruciating pain for the patient. It will be necessary to take a few simple X rays to rule out possibilities of fractures and dislocations of the spine that could cause serious complications. Later, when the severe pain subsides, a series of X rays can be taken in all areas.

Heat, of course, is one of the best treatments for muscle spasms and strains, particularly moist hot packs, which can be placed around the muscles of the neck. This has a very soothing effect. Heat anywhere in the body will promote circulation, and when muscles are torn and bruised, increased circulation can help overcome pain.

In whiplash treatments the neck can be made immobile by wearing a collar, made of either plastic or felt and covered with a soft cloth material. This is called a Thomas collar. However, I have found that excessive wearing of a collar can cause the patient to become overly dependent upon it. After several weeks, when the collar is removed, the patient may feel like his head will fall off without it. For this reason, I advise whiplash victims, even in the beginning, to go without a collar, unless there are compelling medical reasons for wearing one.

Ultrasound treatments, which are simply high frequency sound waves, can overcome muscle spasms and are painless. They are given by physical therapists either in a physician's office or in a hospital. In addition, acupuncture has helped many whiplash patients. Especially when the pain is intense, a series of needles placed in a strategic position may overcome the severe pain. The ratio of those helped is about the same as in the use of acupuncture in other types of cases—about one in four.

The use of medication in overcoming muscle spasm in whiplash injury is far from perfect. Patients too often receive an excessive amount of drugs, especially tranquilizers. These tend to make a patient dopey, and the results often do not justify the side effects. The pain can best be relieved by physical measures and a generous use of standard painkillers, such as aspirin or Tylenol.

Injections into trigger points of pain can also be effective if done by an expert who can locate the painful points. Injections of local anesthetics with hydrocortisone have helped many whiplash patients.

How to Help Yourself If You Sustain a Whiplash Injury

The best treatment for whiplash injury is, of course, prevention. In these days of jammed streets and highways, this is not always easy. One can drive safely and carefully but still be at the mercy of one's fellow drivers. Driving in today's traffic is a tense situation at best. Frustrations, nervousness, and distraction all contribute to the possibility of rear-end collisions with resulting whiplash injuries. All this means that you must drive defensively as well as safely. You should never drive a car without protecting yourself in these ways:

• Always wear seat belts and shoulder straps. Statistics show that their value in a collision is overwhelming.

• Don't tailgate. Leave a generous amount of space between yourself and the car in front of you. A car's length for each ten miles of speed you are driving is the general rule given, but this may not be enough. Bad weather, poor visibility, wet street, and other conditions can affect this rule. Bad brakes and inattention also play a major role in rear-end collisions.

• Care in driving and a well-maintained car may prevent you from tailgating someone else, but what about the driver behind you? As best that you can, you must think for him, too. Be alert, watching the car behind you as well as the one in front of you. That's why your car is equipped with a rear-view mirror.

• If you see someone approaching too fast from the rear, there is a possibility you can quickly pull out into an adjoining lane. If not, you may be able to minimize the possibility of whiplash injury by bracing yourself.

If in spite of all precautions you do have an accident that results in whiplash injury, then what do you do? If you are properly strapped in, there is much less chance of losing consciousness by striking the windshield or being thrown against the roof of the car. So at the moment of impact do not panic. Try to tell yourself that you have come through your ordeal in the best possible shape.

You'll probably have terrible pains in the back of your neck. Your first frantic thought will be that you've broken your neck. Considering the pain you're in, this is a reasonable thought. But if you were strapped in properly and your car is equipped with a head rest to prevent your head from snapping back after being thrown forward, there is an excellent chance that your neck muscles are only strained or torn.

This is painful enough but can be handled. If you find yourself in this predicament, don't under any circumstances twist your neck or let anyone else twist it when they come to help you. In the absence of a regular cervical collar, it is a good idea to have a towel or sweater folded and wrapped around your neck for support. But when you are moved onto an ambulance stretcher, make sure that no one bends your neck. Trained technicians, of course, understand the need for care in handling a whiplash injury. However, if several cars collide at once, victims may get amateur help before the arrival of professional assistance.

If you do have a neck injury, I suggest that you ask to see a specialist in orthopedics or neurosurgery as soon as you arrive at the hospital. The neck, you know, is the channel through which the spinal cord furnishes impulses to the brain. Injury to the neck may involve more than just torn muscles. It may involve the nerves themselves. This could be a very serious matter, and tests by a nerve specialist should be made as soon as possible.

Probably the best advice of all is not to walk away from the scene of an accident, even when you think there is nothing wrong with you. The next day you may find that there are a lot of aches and pains in the back of your head and neck. Your throat may feel sore and your voice may squeak.

This delayed reaction is not unusual. After an accident muscular aches and pains may occur as much as twenty-four hours later. Any weekend gardener or football player will tell you that he feels his worst on Monday morning.

When such pains do occur later, you can apply moist heat at home. Soak a Turkish towel in hot water and apply it to the painful areas. The major precaution here is not to burn yourself. After using these hot packs, try a gentle massage with some alcohol or skin lotion to help relieve the acute muscle spasm that is causing your pain.

When you find a condition of this kind developing after an accident, you can expect to have severe pain for several days. After you have used hot packs and a gentle massage to relieve the spasm as much as possible, by all means consult your family doctor. I have not only seen many patients with this type of injury but I have also been the victim of a minor whiplash injury myself. I can assure you that the symptoms are real and painful.

The severe pain along the back of the neck, or on either side of the neck and the back of the head, comes from irritation of the nerve roots that were stretched when the neck muscles snapped forward and backward so violently. There is no magic treatment for this. It takes time and careful application of the physical measures I described earlier.

Some Disturbing Symptoms That May Follow Whiplash Injury

Extreme nervousness, irritability, and dizziness may occur after a whiplash injury. Doctors once thought that these symptoms had a psychologic or psychosomatic basis. Whiplash injury is caused by torn or strained muscles and sometimes by displaced vertebrae. Therefore, it seemed illogical that dizziness and extreme nervousness should result other than for psychologic reasons. However, there is now enough documentation to make us understand that irritability is due to the bruising of muscles. The dizziness follows from irritation of the special nerves that go to the balance center in the head. Extreme nervousness always follows when a person feels irritable and dizzy.

We also know that a mild concussion often occurs at the time of a whiplash injury, which can also explain irritability and dizziness. Electroencephalograms—brain wave tests—of patients who have sustained recent whiplash injuries have confirmed this diagnosis. A slowing of the brain wave provides objective evidence of a concussion.

Another disturbing symptom is that pain may radiate into the shoulders and arms. When this happens on the left side of the body, it can be extremely frightening to an older person, for it is often mistaken for an angina type pain associated with heart trouble. Many times a victim's blood pressure will shoot up at the moment of whiplash injury. Also an unrelated coronary spasm may occur at the same time, but most of the time the radiation of pain from the shoulder into the left arm can be explained without implicating a heart attack. It is usually the result of irritation caused from bruised nerve roots at the time of the whiplash injury. These symptoms may be prolonged and may not respond to many months of treatment. A thorough medical examination will dispel the normal fear that the pain is from a heart attack.

Some Do's and Don'ts for Whiplash Injury Victims

• Always see a doctor. Don't rely on a quick visit to an emergency room immediately after the accident. Be sure and see your own doctor and allow him to follow your progress for at least ten days to two weeks, which will cover any delayed complaints that may develop.

• Listen to your doctor's advice and get plenty of rest. This means taking time away from work or household duties. This enforced rest interrupts the patient's normal routine of life and accounts for many of the psychologic problems that follow this type of injury.

• Expect a prolonged period of discomfort if you have severe complaints at the initial time of injury. You can't rush getting well, for there is no shortcut.

• Forget about the well-meaning neighbor who will either scare you to death with horror tales of what happened to his cousin or will give you the wrong advice on how to cure yourself.

• If you possibly can, don't talk about your accident. The more you talk about it, the more harm it will do you. It revives in your mind the possibility that you might have been killed, restimulates irritation over how much damage was done to your car, and revives resentment toward the driver responsible for your condition. All of these irritations and resentments are road blocks to your recovery. It is not easy to listen to someone who says, "Forget it." But you should discipline yourself to do just that if you can. Believe me, it will be a genuine help in your recovery.

• If you are injured in a whiplash accident caused by another driver, you can expect insurance companies to take a great interest in you and your condition. After all, they have considerable money at stake. So don't get overly upset by their demands for continual examinations by company doctors. This is a normal course of procedure after an accident. They may, of course, try to limit the seriousness of your injury.

• Don't accept surgical treatment for your pain without the opinions of several specialists. I am not speaking of emergency surgery for a dislocated neck injury. In such a case, there is danger of paralysis, and an operation on the spine is definitely indicated. But in the case of an elective operation— that is, one planned to relieve pain—great care must be taken before you submit to this type of operation. In the last twenty years neurosurgeons and orthopedic surgeons have been enthusiastic about fusion operations of the cervical spine (neck area). But results in this area have not been successful in more than 60 percent of cases. I suggest that you make sure you get the opinion of several experts in the field before undergoing an operation of this type.

• An injury of this type means different things to different people. A concert pianist would view a whiplash injury as a major catastrophe, for it would prevent him from giving concerts. On the other hand, a short-order cook might not be so overwhelmed by his injury. In other words, each of us places a personal value on what our physical performance means to us and how an accident limits the performance of our work and activity. Consequently, our mental attitude varies considerably and can intensify our suffering. The prescription here is simple: Accept your condition and don't worry about it. Unfortunately, too many find this medicine difficult or impossible to take.

Summary

If you are the victim of a whiplash injury, don't panic. Remember that the chances are in your favor that the injury is restricted to bruising muscles and joints in your neck.

There is no magic treatment for this type of injury. Just make sure that you go to a hospital for a careful evaluation. When moved from the scene of the accident, try to control movements of your neck. A towel wrapped around your neck will help to prevent excessive movement, and you can also place both of your hands behind your neck to guard against any jolts as you are moved. If you are taken to an emergency room, make sure you are given a soft cervical collar. And, if possible, consult your doctor the very next morning. If there is any doubt about your condition, stay in the hospital and take the advice of the doctors in the emergency room. Pain may persist for several months. There is no quick way to recovery. It is all a matter of time.

10

NEURALGIA
AND NEURITIS:
FACE, HEAD, CHEST

Up to now I have been talking about conditions where nerves
have been compressed or irritated to create pain. I would like
to explain a different type of pain caused by trouble in the
nerve itself. This pain comes from either of two conditions
known as *neuritis* or *neuralgia.*

As I explained earlier, *itis* means inflammation or irritation. *Appendicitis* means an inflamed appendix and *laryn-
gitis* is a sore throat, often caused by bacterial infections in
the back of the throat. *Neuritis*, then, means an inflammation of a nerve, and *neuralgia* refers to a painful nerve.
Sometimes these medical terms are interchanged.

The condition called neuritis has been associated with
diabetes, lead poisoning, exposure to arsenic, and lack of
vitamins B and C. The neuralgic condition still baffles us. We
have no cause, specifically identified, to explain neuralgia.
Many times we use the word to identify a condition in the
face or head when we have no specific cause to explain the
severe pain. The one exception is a virus, such as the cold
sore virus that causes lip blister. It may attack the nerve root
in the face, head, or chest to produce a herpes or vesicle
(blister) formation. This condition often results in a severe
neuralgic pain both during and following the blister period.

One of the worst types of neuralgic pain is facial neuralgia or trigeminal neuralgia, so-called because it affects the large trigeminal nerve that supplies the face from the forehead to the chin. This condition is often associated with severe spasm of the face.

Ruth was seventy and a grandmother several times over but hardly looked it, for she enjoyed remarkably good health. For Ruth, these were truly the golden years, and she kept busy sewing, cooking, playing the piano, and enjoying life with her recently retired husband. Then suddenly the dark cloud of neuralgic pain intruded upon her happiness. She first felt it as a severe shooting pain in the eye and over the right part of the forehead.

Describing the pain later, she said, "I felt like my eyeball had exploded like a firecracker. The pain seemed to last for hours, and I was surprised when I looked at the clock. Only a few seconds had passed."

After several more attacks Ruth went to see an eye doctor. He found nothing in the eye to cause the attacks. He suggested that she see her medical doctor for a complete checkup. This she dutifully did. The family doctor gave her an examination but also found nothing wrong.

Then one day the pain struck while she was playing the piano. It was so intense that she almost fell off the piano stool. This time the pain spasm lasted a full minute and kept recurring every several hours. She returned to her doctor, who, now suspecting neuralgia, recommended that she see a nerve specialist.

Ruth's examination showed no abnormal neurological signs, by which I mean that the movement of her face and the feeling over her forehead, cheek, and jaw were all within normal limits. There was no evidence of any tumor pressing on her brain or on the trigeminal nerve in the face.

She interrupted the examination to ask anxiously, "Doctor, you can do something for me, can't you? No one can find anything wrong. I know they think it's just my nerves. But there *is* something wrong. I couldn't just imagine anything as terrible as these pains."

"I'm sure we can help you," the doctor replied soothingly. "So far we have found out what isn't wrong, and that's progress in itself. And I agree that your trouble isn't nerves, but I think we'll find it in a nerve.

"Now in your face," he went on, "there is a trigeminal nerve that splits into three parts. One goes to the forehead. Another goes to the cheek, and the third part goes into the tongue and the lower jaw. Since your pain is over your eye, there is a strong possibility that you have neuralgia in the first division of the trigeminal nerve." Trigeminal neuralgia—Ruth's case—is an irritation of the fifth cranial nerve.

"Is there anything you can do about it?" she asked anxiously.

"First we must find out if this diagnosis is correct," he replied. "So let's try this. . . ."

His fingers began to trace a pattern across her forehead just above the eyebrow. Then he began tapping over the eyebrow at the position where the first division of the trigeminal nerve exits from the skull.

Suddenly Ruth almost doubled up with pain. Her face twisted in agony, and the pain area reddened. The doctor reached quickly for a syringe and injected a local anesthetic into the painful area.

The pain disappeared as the anesthetic took effect. "That's it!" she cried. "That's just how it felt before."

With the diagnosis verified, the doctor then advised Ruth to let him inject a few drops of alcohol into the nerve. He assured her that this would relieve any future pain for about eighteen months. The effect of the alcohol injection would wear off in that time, he explained, but they could hope that the neuralgia condition would correct itself by then. If not, then he would attack the problem from another angle.

He went on to explain that the alcohol injection would block the nerve entirely. Her face, in the area served by the first division of the trigeminal nerve, would be numb as long as the alcohol injection was effective. Ruth preferred numbness to the excruciating pain, and the injection was performed.

This is a classic case of trigeminal neuralgia. Today, most neurologists who see this condition start their patients off on new drugs such as Tegretol. However, these drugs must be given under careful supervision of a physician, for they can cause some bad effects on the blood. Dilantin is another drug that has been used with some success. Still another treatment used for many years is the injection of vitamin B_{12} in large amounts.

Drugs of this type were not used in Ruth's case because her pain was localized to the first division and was easily accessible to an alcohol injection.

I think that it is better to inject the nerve when it is accessible rather than start a patient on drugs. One injection of a few drops of alcohol can numb the affected area sufficiently to relieve pain for a year to eighteen months. Then, drugs can be used if the pain reoccurs.

Some Other Types of Facial Neuralgia

In addition to neuralgias of the face, there is another type that affects the back of the throat in the tonsillar area. This is called *glossopharyngeal neuralgia*, because it is an irritation of the glossopharyngeal or ninth cranial nerve.

Another common neuralgia in the head is the *occipital*. This is a shooting pain that goes from a region about one inch behind the back of the ear and shoots over the top of the head. This type of neuralgia can follow a whiplash injury, but it often comes on without any history of a previous injury. It can be helped by an injection into the region of the greater occipital (back of the skull) nerve.

Surgical Treatment for Neuralgia

The alcohol injection treatment for neuralgia, unfortunately, is not always a cure. This treatment controls the pain for twelve to eighteen months. Then the nerve regenerates itself, and a second injection is not as effective as the first. Therefore, it is sometimes necessary when the pain reoccurs to advise surgical treatment, and the nerve can then be cut. This is done by making a fine incision above the eyebrow, in the case of trigeminal neuralgia, or in the occipital nerve in the back of the head to relieve occipital neuralgia.

Pain sometimes reoccurs after cutting the nerve. Then, a deeper operation has to be performed. This procedure, done by a neurological surgeon, is one of the early triumphs in the history of neurosurgery. The operation was very popular until ten years ago, when newer drugs, such as Tegretol, became available. Nevertheless, surgery is still the primary hope for patients who get no relief from the newer drugs or who develop bad reactions to these drugs. The operation is done today with greater precision than ever by using a surgical microscope.

The drawback to any of these surgical treatments is that all of them result in numbness over the area of the face supplied by the treated nerve. This numbness compares to the way your lip feels after it has been deadened with Novocain by a dentist. It is very annoying to many people. However, most patients who have been through the absolute agony of neuralgic attacks welcome any kind of relief. I have never seen a patient refuse surgical treatment once other measures have failed.

Acupuncture for Trigeminal Neuralgia

The Chinese claim that trigeminal neuralgia pains can be greatly relieved by acupuncture. Experience in the United States is limited. I have tried this type of treatment in patients with trigeminal neuralgia and have helped some of them over an acute attack. But at this time I have no statistics in favor of or against acupuncture. Certainly it should be tried, for it is safe and a relatively simple procedure.

Summary of Treatment for Trigeminal Neuralgia

If you experience a recurrence of pains in your face that last just a few minutes, then neuralgia is the most likely diagnosis. If the pain lasts for hours, then it is not a true trigeminal neuralgia. The trouble is caused by something else. Your doctor, of course, is the one to make this precise diagnosis. It is a condition that does not show any abnormal findings or outward signs. So you must be able to give the doctor a precise history of how long the pain lasts and how it occurs.

This condition is often mistaken for toothache, so one good piece of advice is not to let a dentist extract all your teeth. First see your doctor and a neurological specialist to be sure.

The following is a summary of the different treatments:

DRUGS

In the last ten years drugs like Dilantin and more recently Tegretol have been used with increasing success to control this type of pain. Tranquilizers have also been used to control the nervousness that occurs as a result of the unpredictable pain. However, narcotics must be avoided. They cannot help you, and there is danger of addiction.

ACUPUNCTURE

The jury is not in yet on this one. It is a simple and safe technique. It has helped in some cases and is certainly worth trying.

INJECTION TECHNIQUES

Temporary destruction of the nerve with alcohol injections is still the simplest method of controlling the pain for a limited time. The blocked nerve will regenerate itself after a year to eighteen months. And as I noted earlier, a second nerve block is not as helpful as the first.

NEWER SURGICAL METHODS

In recent years there has been a trend to take advantage of the X-ray television technique. This permits a needle to be placed into the base of the skull where the nerve center for the trigeminal nerve is located. Then the nerve center can be destroyed with safety by the use of radio-frequency current. This method is encouraging and has enabled neurosurgeons to avoid major operations. As in all such treatments for neuralgia, numbness over the affected area will be a consequence, but there are few other complications.

NERVE STIMULATION TECHNIQUES

Some years ago Dr. William Sweet of the Harvard Medical School conceived the idea of stimulating the nerves of the face to overcome trigeminal pain. He introduced a fine wire electrode stimulator that can be placed into the nerve at its exit from the cheekbone. He claims this type of technique can temporarily control pain without producing numbness. This is part of the newer counterirritation techniques still under development to avoid a nerve destruction to overcome pain.

Neuralgias of the Chest Masquerading as Heart Attacks

While my previous discussions have involved neuralgias of the face, you can have this condition in other parts of the body as well. For example, Oscar, a forty-seven-year-old accountant, was stricken with a severe pain over the left side of his chest. He was rushed to the hospital in the early morning hours, and subsequent tests showed that he did not have a heart condition. He returned to work, for he was the hard-driving type who did not like to baby himself. His pains continued to reoccur, coming from his spine around the left side of his chest. The continuous pain convinced him that he was having a heart spasm. His physician reassured him many times that this was not so, as did an outstanding heart specialist. The heart specialist, suspecting neuritis, sent Oscar to a neurosurgeon, who found that the patient had a neuritis of the nerves that originate under the ribs. These are called the intercostal nerves. Further studies revealed that Oscar was a borderline diabetic, and the final diagnosis was that his pain was a mild diabetic neuritis.

Oscar was greatly relieved to learn that he definitely did not have a heart condition. He was reluctant to undergo surgery to correct his condition, but when he did not get better, an operation was performed to cut the nerves, and he is now completely free of severe attacks of pain.

Oscar's case points out a very important fact. We have become accustomed to thinking of a pain over the chest as indicating a heart attack. There are many other conditions that can cause these same symptoms. This is why medicine—and especially pain control—is an art rather than a science.

Trigger Points

A very common condition is myositis, an irritation of the muscles themselves. Muscles, after all, are living structures, and they can become irritated or bruised. The resulting painful muscles then act as trigger points to refer pain to other areas. The term *trigger point* is used because just as pulling the trigger of a gun sends a bullet off in a direction, the pushing or irritation of a muscles in, say, the wing of the shoulder blade, can shoot pain off into the arm itself.

A very disturbing type of trigger point pain can originate in the shoulder girdle. Sometimes the trigger can be in the shoulder girdle muscles and shoot into the left arm. Application of heat or an injection into the trigger point area will relieve such pain. Some patients, especially tense and anxious ones, can develop a series of trigger points. These can occur over the shoulders, the front of the chest, and over the abdomen.

Neuritis and Alcohol

Excessive intake of alcohol not only destroys the liver but can affect the nerves as well. There is a condition called alcoholic neuritis, which consists of shooting pains in the arms and legs of people who drink excessively, especially without eating properly. I know a patient who would drink for several weeks without eating. He developed such severe shooting pains in his arms and legs that they almost drove him crazy. He was relieved by an intake of proper vitamins and a proper diet.

The lack of vitamin B has been known to cause neuralgic and neuritic pains, but it is rare to see these conditions in our society where most people have an abundance of food. One of the classic conditions of vitamin deficiency is beriberi. It was the study of this wasting disease that led to the discovery of vitamin B as essential for healthy nerves. By *nerves* I do not mean emotional control but the actual structures that control pain in the body.

Neuritis and Diabetes

I do not want to alarm anyone who may have diabetes, but there is an association between diabetes and neuritis. Most diabetics who are careful will not develop neuritis. If it does occur, the condition may often be relieved.

Abdominal Pains That Masquerade as Ulcers and Cancer

Just as a neuritic pain in the chest frightens us with the thought of a heart attack, a severe pain in the stomach fills us with fear of appendicitis or a ruptured ulcer. Fortunately, the abdomen is less prone to neuralgic pains than the chest wall, perhaps because there are more structures in the chest, especially with the movement of respiration, which can become irritated. Also, the nerves that go into the chest wall have to traverse a longer distance. Since there are numerous neuralgic type pains that can mimic conditions in the stomach or guts, a good rule to follow is to have any constant pain in this area checked thoroughly by your doctor.

What to Do If You Have Neuralgia and Neuritis

If you find yourself with sharp shooting pains in your face, as Ruth did, make sure you consult your doctor before concluding that you have the same thing. Don't shop around.

Insist on an examination by a neurological specialist. He has the training and experience to determine if you have a true neuritic condition. In the long run this is the quickest way to get help.

If you are a diabetic, don't play games with yourself. Follow your doctor's advice and maintain a careful control of your diabetes. Make sure that you take an extra amount of vitamin B daily as insurance against diabetic neuritis. You might also refrain from excessive alcohol and avoid fatigue, both of which can promote neuralgia and neuritis.

Today there are various ways to attack neuralgia and neuritis, so do not be too hasty about agreeing to an operation for the destruction of nerves. Get the opinions of several specialists. An operation may be necessary, but try the simpler methods first. If you need surgery, make sure the neurosurgeon is certified by the American Board of Neurological Surgery, which you can easily do by consulting the *Directory of Medical Specialists* in your public library.

11

PELVIC PAINS
IN WOMEN

The special anatomy of a woman predisposes her to have certain complaints in her pelvic organs. An understanding of the inside of a woman's pelvis may explain some of these complaints, such as painful menstruation with crampy sensations or a tightness and painful aching in the pelvic structures or vagina.

The female pelvis houses the vagina and its attached uterus or womb. These structures are located between the urinary bladder in front of the uterus and the rectum behind it. Attached to the uterus, which is a pear-shaped muscular organ that opens into the vagina below it, are two tubes that hang like stems of a flower to the uterus. These are the Fallopian tubes and beneath them are attached two vital structures called ovaries, which are shaped like almonds.

Normally, every twenty-eight days the ovaries will produce a female egg or ovum. This egg must break through the wall of the ovary and pass through the Fallopian tube inwardly to the uterus or womb. If the egg is not fertilized at this time by a male sperm deposited in the vagina, the ovum will not find a prepared layer in the uterus for its growth. Consequently, the ovum will be expelled along with the built-up layers in the inner lining of the uterus. When this happens, a bloody discharge takes place for four to five days. This is called a monthly flow or menstruation, from the Latin word *mensis*, meaning month. The ancients knew of this cycle of monthly blood flow and could almost time the calendar by it.

The ovum is discharged in about the midcycle or about the fourteenth day. At the moment of expulsion from the ovary a pain may take place. This can be a severe cramp, colorfully described by the Germans as *mittelschmertz*, or middle pain.

Painful Menstruation

Why is it that some women will complain more than others about a painful monthly flow? The case of Rosalie might give a clue to one possibility. From her first menstruation at the age of twelve, Rosalie complained of a crampy sensation and such discomfort that she had to miss school for several days. The situation did not improve with time. All her life she dreaded the coming of her monthly period. When I questioned her about the background of her trouble, she admitted that her mother had made a great fuss over Rosalie's first menstruation.

"She told me I was going to bleed down there and not to fail to let her know when it happened," Rosalie said. "When it did, she put me to bed and sat with me to comfort me. She said she knew how terrible I felt and not to be shocked by the blood."

Rosalie related that a hot water bottle was placed over her lower abdomen and she was given some aspirin. In every way she was made to feel that she was genuinely sick. Later, when she tried to cut herself free from her mother's control, she still found that her periods were painful. During the early years of her marriage she tried bravely to hide her misery from her husband.

Finally, she decided to seek medical help in overcoming her abnormal fear of menstruation. A complete medical examination showed no abnormality in her vaginal structure. For that matter, she had never complained of pain during intercourse. The examination, revealing no abnormality, relieved her. She was then slowly able to overcome her fear. In time, with the help of her doctor and a considerate husband, she was able to reduce her discomfort from five days to about one day of mild pain.

You will probably conclude that Rosalie's dysmenorrhea, or painful monthly flow, was mainly mental or emotional. I must admit that she did develop an abnormal behavior reaction from her mother's frightening attitude. Other girls who are taught not to pay much attention to the discomfort of a monthly flow seem to get along quite well.

However, there are times when a physical disturbance can be responsible for menstruation pain. I remember a charming patient named Barbara who was almost driven wild by cramping sensations during her monthly flow. She was told that her distress was all emotional. She listened, did her best to convince herself that it was all in her mind, but her monthly pain did not go away. She finally consulted a good gynecologist who found that her pelvic structures were not quite normal. She apparently had a very narrow vaginal opening and the normal hymen had not completely ruptured. This caused a backing up of blood, which produced considerable pain. She was relieved by corrective surgery.

How You Can Help Yourself If You Have Pelvic Pain

Why not make a checklist as to how you have been feeling each month? Use a calendar to list how you felt before the monthly flow, during, and after it. By checking this, you may find some relationship between your discomfort and other events in your life.

Think hard on how you first learned about your monthly flow. Was your mother very attentive? Did she seem to baby you or overprotect you? Did she try to make you feel that there was nothing to it when you felt you needed help? Were you accustomed to taking aspirin or some other pain-killing drug during this time? Did your monthly flow change if you took birth control pills? After you have analyzed yourself, why not consult a good family doctor and, if necessary, a gynecologist?

Another type of pelvic pain is that which occurs during intercourse. Most women are extremely reticent about talking to a doctor about this. Really, there is nothing to be ashamed of. I am sure you will agree that intercourse is a normal function. If you are having pain during the act, or even afterward, instead of refraining, why not come out in the open and tell your partner that it is painful. He will probably agree that complete physical evaluation is in order. Sometimes a simple technique of proper lubrication is sufficient to overcome pain.

Some Simple Techniques of Obtaining Relief from Pelvic Pain

Some women have told me that a mild sitz bath before the monthly flow seems to help them. This is easy to do. You can buy a sitz bathtub that fits on top of the toilet seat. If the water is kept warm but not scalding, sitting in it for about ten minutes will greatly aid in relieving pelvic congestion and pain. If you prefer sitting in a shallow tub of water, that is fine also, but if you have enough time to get into a full tub of water—comfortably warm—you will find complete relief most of the time. A sitz bath is also a good technique to relieve pain that may happen after intercourse. Just sit in a warm sitz bath and you will get relief in about twenty minutes.

If the sitz bath doesn't help, and you know that this type of pain is regular, why not take a couple of aspirin before the period starts and maintain this each day? It is also important to drink plenty of liquids and to allow yourself extra rest during this period.

Constipation is also an enemy of freedom from pelvic pain. Make sure you do not allow yourself to become constipated. Keep your bowels open with plenty of fresh fruit and establish proper times for elimination.

How Your Doctor May Help You

Suppose you have painful menstruation, pain during intercourse, and other pains in and around your pelvic regions. You are terribly worried, and rightly so. Such pains are not normal, and this area should not be a source of discomfort to you.

First, you should see your doctor and insist upon a complete examination. Sometimes the trouble may be a persistent discharge from the vagina, causing considerable irritation and pain. A common cause of this condition is a fungus infection. This can be treated with some newer drugs.

Trouble may also be caused by sagging muscles. So your doctor may teach you some basic exercises to strengthen your pelvic wall: A simple one prescribed is to try and walk on all fours. Another is to tighten the muscles of your pelvic wall. A mild sedative at night will help you get proper rest and with it control of discomfort.

What about Surgical Treatment

Any type of surgical treatment for control of pelvic pain should be undertaken with extreme caution. I am, of course, assuming that you have undergone a complete examination and that no tumor has been found and that suspicion of cancer has been ruled out by the Papanicolaou stain, commonly known as the Pap test. The latter technique is a staining of cells from the cervix, which is that part of the uterus that connects with the roof of the vagina.

Every woman should have a Papanicolaou stain yearly. This can be done simply and safely, and it rules out any danger of undetected cancer of the cervix.

For patients with persistent menstrual pain or dysmenorrhea, an operation called *presacral neurectomy* became popular several years ago. This operation consists of cutting those nerves that go to the posterior or back wall of the pelvis. This type of operation has to be done with extreme caution and should not be accepted without the opinions of several doctors.

Some Final Thoughts

Just remember that pelvic pains, especially those that arise during the menstrual cycle, can be controlled with common sense. In all cases women have been helped by reassurance that comes from a complete examination and simple techniques such as a sitz bath at the time of the period.

12

NEW HOPE FOR RELIEF FROM PAIN FOR CANCER VICTIMS

I had just come from Mary Ann's hospital room. As I walked down the hospital corridor, I was thinking about how bravely this forty-seven-year-old, once vivacious woman had tried to smile despite the unbearable pain in her right hip. I paused to look out the window at the gray, drizzling rain as I tried to form the words I would have to give her waiting husband.

For a year Mary Ann had had spotty vaginal bleeding, which she had neglected. She had been in excruciating pain for the past three months, but she hoped it would disappear. In the course of an examination, her family doctor discovered that she had cancer of the womb and that the cancerous growth had spread into the right side of her pelvis. Her intense pain was coming from irritation of the nerves in her right leg. Because of it she was referred for pain control.

I broke the news to her husband, Don, as gently as I could. He took it much harder than his wife had. I explained that we would have a specialist in cobalt treatment see her. If this failed to bring her relief, then I was sure she could be helped by a new neurosurgical procedure. This brought him some comfort. I can still remember his words: "Doctor, I know how serious cancer is, especially after it has spread, as hers has. If she can't be cured, then I beg you, doctor, please don't let her suffer. She's such a wonderful person. If she has to die, I don't want her to suffer the rest of her life the way she is suffering now."

How often I have heard similar words from the families of patients in extreme pain. Sometimes I have been implored to put a patient out of his misery. I can only answer such requests: "I'm sorry, but I took an oath to preserve life. I will do what I can to relieve the pain for your loved one."

The reply most often was, "Doctor, I don't expect miracles, and I know that mercy killing is out of the question. But please promise me that you will do everything possible to make the last days bearable."

What You Can Do to Help If You Suspect Cancer

What can be done to make life bearable for someone with incurable cancer? So much has been written about cancer and its danger signals that I see no purpose in repeating it here. By now almost every educated person knows that bleeding when vomiting or coughing, or bleeding from the rectum during a bowel movement may be a sign of cancer.

Pain, unfortunately, is not the earliest indication of cancer. The pain—and it can be excruciating—comes after the disease invades tissues where there are abundant nerves— places like the covering of bones or nerves that exit from the spinal cord; areas along the angle of the jaw, deep in the neck, the hip, anywhere along the chest; or in the abdomen. This underscores the great value of pain as a signal that something is wrong. If cancer produced immediate pain, diagnosis would be quick and in most cases could be cured. But once the cancer spreads to the point where pain is a problem, the best we can do is to recognize its reality and do what we can to ease the discomfort.

So the first important step in controlling cancer pain is to make the initial diagnosis. Seeing your doctor at the first sign of the normal danger signals is still step number one.

Let us say that you have received a diagnosis of cancer. This does not necessarily mean that you have to dread a future of unbearable pain. Today we can diagnose many types of cancer in their early stages, when there is a good chance of treating them successfully.

Of course, there are cases like Mary Ann. Unfortunately, she did not consult a doctor early enough, when she saw that blood was coming from her vagina. Why she waited, I do not know. She may have thought that she was approaching change of life earlier than expected, assuming that the bleeding was part of the change. Instead of visiting a gynecologist for a Papanicolaou test, which would have detected cancer of the cervix of her uterus, she kept putting it off. Radium and cobalt therapy might have controlled the disease in the beginning. The radiotherapist felt her case was too advanced for X-ray therapy, so I performed a procedure called cordotomy, which is a selective cutting of certain nerve pathways in the spinal cord.

Once you have had an early diagnosis of cancer and treatment given, your chances of having to suffer extreme pain are fortunately in the minority. The actual statistics of persistent pain are not known to us. Maybe 5 to 10 percent of patients will have intractable pain, and even this group can be helped by neurosurgical techniques.

How Doctors Help to Relieve Cancer Pain

As I have suggested, precise diagnosis is the most important part of cancer treatment. Diagnosis is much easier today than it was in the past. We now have atomic tests, which can be done with relative safety, that can graphically pick up cancers almost anywhere in the body.

Before World War II, we relied almost exclusively on X rays. An X ray is good for detecting trouble in bones but less so in tissues. Today, we have atomic particle techniques that can help detect cancer in the brain, known as the brain scan technique. Another method to detect cancer is radioactive scanning of the bones. More recently the methods of radar have been passed on to the physician and used as a diagnostic tool in the form of ultrasonography. This technique sends a beam of sound to a depth of the body and bounces it back to measure the location and type of cancer masses in various portions of the abdomen. In this manner, a large tumor can be visualized even in such hidden places as the liver or the pancreas.

Contrast X-ray studies have been available for years and were recently improved by the development of X-ray television. A catheter, which is a wormlike tube, can be inserted into a major blood vessel in the groin and dye can be injected. This will help to demonstrate cancer masses in various parts of the kidneys, liver, or bowels. The same dye can be injected into the cerebral blood vessels to make evident various types of brain tumors. Such techniques are called *angiograms*, and they provide ways to make precise, safe, and early diagnoses of cancer.

Some Forms of Cancer Treatment

Anti-cancer drugs have become more available in the last fifteen years. Unfortunately, we do not have a vaccine or specific drug for cancer. Recently, there was a breakthrough discovery for a certain type of leukemia in children, which gives hope for the development of specific cancer drugs in the future.

The cobalt treatment employs radiation. The use of the cobalt form of radiotherapy allows the cancer therapist or the treating physician to deliver high doses of radiation to smaller targets, permitting a greater and safer destruction of tumor tissues without also destroying healthy tissues.

Some New Techniques for Relief of Cancer Pain

Neurosurgeons have pioneered in the relief of cancer pain through their ability to operate on the nervous system. In fact, some of the early triumphs in neurosurgery dealt with pain relief. In the first decades of the twentieth century the operation of cordotomy was developed in Philadelphia by Drs. William Spiller and Charles Frazier. These two physicians were instrumental in developing to a high point not only the operation for relief of facial pain but also the cordotomy operation in the spinal cord to relieve unbearable pain secondary to cancer.

For almost fifty years the cordotomy operation was the mainstay of neurosurgical procedures to relieve pain in cancer patients. This particular operation consists of opening the spinal canal, generally in the area between the shoulder blades or in the cervical spine beneath the base of the head. The opening is made by laminectomy, which consists of removing bone from the roof of the spinal canal or lamina to expose the spinal cord.

The surgeon then takes delicate instruments and exposes a tiny area in the front of the spinal cord known as the *anterolateral* white column. It is known to neurosurgeons that pain in the left hip travels in the spinal cord on the *right* side. For reasons unknown, the pain fibers that serve the left hip, in this example, travel up the right side of the spinal cord, performing a crossover.

Moreover, these fibers bind together in a precise area, no

larger than a pea. This area is exposed by the laminectomy, and an incision is made with a fine surgical blade or cataract-type knife. The depth of the incision is not more than a six-teenth of an inch deep. Once this is done, there is a loss of perception of painful stimuli from a pin prick in the opposite side of the body. The patient also loses perception of hot and cold. So if the cordotomy is performed between the shoulder blades, the result will be a numbness of the entire left side from the toe almost to the nipple of the breast. This will relieve permanently unbearable pain from cancer in the left hip, as in Mary Ann's case.

In 1963 an imaginative neurosurgeon named Sean Mullan, at the University of Chicago, made a major contribution to pain control. Mullan took advantage of advancements in X-ray television and three-dimensional or stereotaxic neuro-surgery to perform a cordotomy without a laminectomy. He first used a strontium probe. Then later he developed a tech-nique of guiding a fine electric wire through a needle into the anterolateral portion of the spinal cord—that is, the area where the pain-bearing pathways are normally cut by the surgeon's knife. Once this fine wire is directed into the pain-bearing pathways, the area can be disconnected by a special apparatus known as a radio-frequency generator. Actually, this innovation was made by Dr. Hubert Rosomoff, profes-sor of neurosurgery at the University of Miami. It produces waves of the same frequency as radio. This energy destroys the pain-bearing pathways with great safety.

The value of the stereotaxic—or percutaneous cordot-omy—developed by Dr. Mullan is this: Patients with unbear-able pain of cancer can be relieved of their agony without an open operation. This means that thousands of patients who previously had refused cordotomy because of its magnitude now have hope of spending their final months of life without pain. Treatment is much like going to a dentist. That is, the patient is given a local anesthesia and made comfortable on a special X-ray television operating room table, while the pain-bearing pathway is localized safely, then disconnected. I have been greatly impressed by the relative simplicity of this procedure, even though it requires more skill to do than an "open" operation. The Mullan stereotaxic cordotomy is a triumph of modern technology.

There is another operation that neurosurgeons have developed within the past twenty years to relieve unbearable cancer pain. This is to disconnect the higher centers of the brain. In the forward part of the brain there are two areas known as the *cingulate gyri*. These are the higher centers for emotional response to pain or disturbing sensations. Through two dime-sized openings into the skull, similar electrodes used for the radio-frequency destruction of the spinal cord are used to disconnect the cingulums. This is done without pain under a local anesthetic because once the skin is incised and the skull opened, there is no pain as the electrical wires find their targets in the brain.

These are some of the newer techniques used by neurosurgeons to relieve the unbearable pain of cancer. Other operations, which I will just touch on, include the removal of the pituitary gland or *hypophysis*. The reason the pituitary gland or hypophysis controls pain is that the gland supports the spread of cancer tissue. Unfortunately, the gland cannot be destroyed by closed methods, except by highly sophisticated X-ray machines, but these are not available in most centers.

Hypophysectomy can by done by placing a special electrode through the roof of the nose. Again, this is done with the patient gently asleep. X-ray television has made this a simple operation, and it can be performed on patients with greatly advanced cancer that has spread to the bones. The basic technique was devised by Dr. Jean Talairach of Paris. This method was modified and then developed to perfection by Dr. Nicholas Zervas in Boston. The open operation of exposing the gland through the nose and removing it with a microscope has found greater usefulness in the hands of neurosurgeons in Montreal, Canada, particularly by Dr. Jules Hardy of the Notre Dame Hospital.

How to Prepare Yourself for Prolonged Suffering and Pain

I have touched upon some of the miracles of neurosurgery to control cancer pain. Unfortunately, scientific control of pain is not the whole story. Associated with agony and suffering is the mental attitude of the dying patient. A psychiatrist named Elisabeth Kübler-Ross made a major contribution in her studies on *Death and Dying,* and I highly recommend her book. She found that patients who are told that they have an incurable disease, such as cancer, often go through several stages. Shock and disbelief is apparently the first stage. Next the patient may try to make "deals," or may go into a phase of severe depression. He tries to make a deal with a higher power by praying, "God, if you'll give me another chance, I'll be better." After this stage passes the patient can then come to a rational approach to the inevitable fate of death.

I have helped many patients by offering them medical relief of pain. After this was done, I tried to help them understand that even a few additional months of life free of pain and suffering has great value to them and to their families. But let's face it. Without a deeper, philosophic and religious outlook, we cannot sustain ourselves in the final months of suffering that accompanies a disease like cancer. The shock is deep and soul-shaking when a patient comes to realize that he has an incurable disease. At that time, he realizes that it is only a question of time before he dies. This thought of predictable death, for which we have no preparation in the contemporary world, must revolt and shock us. It is strange that we are taught so many skills, but we know nothing about preparing to die.

Summary

We like to pride ourselves on being a nation of doers. So our approach to the patient with cancer is to try and do something to help relieve his suffering. The greatest tool we have is early diagnosis. Not all patients with cancer will suffer unbearable pain. The worst pain happens in those whose malignancies have spread into nerve endings. Now even these people can take hope from newer techniques, such as cobalt radiation treatments and new anti-cancer drugs. When these fail to control the pain and check the spread of the cancerous mass, then newer neurological techniques, such as stereotaxic cordotomy and its modifications, are available in all neurological centers. These procedures give sufficient relief so that the patient can forego strong narcotics for many months until death relieves him permanently of all pain. Lastly, a philosophic and religious outlook can be helpful in making terminal pain and suffering bearable.

13

HOW YOU CAN
HELP YOURSELF
FIND RELIEF
FROM PAIN

The medical journal *Postgraduate Medicine*, in May 1973, dedicated an entire issue to pain, in which Dr. John Bonica, an outstanding expert and authority on pain control, estimated that ten billion dollars were spent annually in the control of chronic pain! This says nothing for the hours of endless despair and human misery represented by this tremendous expenditure of money.

We have made great advances in medical science that we can point to with pride. The Salk vaccine has brought polio under control. Insulin aids the diabetic. Antibiotics work against severe infection, and hopeful new cures loom on the horizon for cancer and even hardening of the arteries. Yet the scourge of chronic pain is still with us, not amenable to an easy solution. We can do a lot for it, and there is definitely new hope for chronic sufferers today. However, pain will not be brought under total control until we understand the intricate workings of our computerlike nervous systems.

So each of us must understand what can be done for us and—equally important—*what we can do for ourselves*. Anyone who has made the rounds of doctors, seeking relief from chronic headaches, backaches, shoulder pains, and the like knows what I am talking about.

We have learned a lot about the nervous system and the pathways that transmit pain through the body. This knowledge permits us to do a lot to alleviate pain, but it is hardly sufficient to explain all we need to know to control it. This knowledge has at least brought us to a more realistic understanding. We no longer try to explain pain in terms of demons invading the body, as did the witch doctors of ancient times. Yet in our vain search for relief, we have adopted the old Chinese technique of acupuncture, hoping we can put a balance in the Yang and Yin that is causing pain. Actually, acupuncture works in a limited way because of counterirritation, a known phenomenon.

The science of psychology is popular today, and new strides in this science bear on control of pain. We have learned that pain sufferers, when the cause is not cancer, can train themselves to raise the thresholds of pain perception through operant conditioning. This means a self-discipline to not give in to pain when it assails us. Actually, this is not a great new advance. We are just going back to an old idea and cloaking it in modern terms. Nevertheless, the attitude toward pain differs in various individuals, and this pain threshold is a key point in helping yourself if you are a victim of chronic pain.

In an earlier chapter I spoke of how doctors find the causes of your pain. There is really no shortcut to this approach. If you take your own pain-killing drugs, you may be hiding a serious illness that could take your life. You will find that seeing your family doctor, a man trained to seek causes, is your best approach. Unfortunately, advice to see your family doctor is not realistic in today's mobile society. The former family doctor himself grew older with a family. He understood them and their physical problems. Today thirty-six million Americans move each year and do not have family physicians. So the next best approach is to seek out a group of doctors who practice in a common setting and let them try to help you find the cause of your pain and its relief. This approach is why, perhaps, the great clinics like Mayo and Lahey and smaller groups of doctors have succeeded and continue to provide good medical care.

Now that you know what can be done for your pain, you will also appreciate the limitations doctors face and will not expect miracles. You will shun the person with quick answers and the quack cures. People in pain waste millions of dollars annually in seeking help from gadgets for massage, useless ointments, and worthless liniments. Federal control of fake medical material is a long way from adequate, and in the backs of cheaper magazines you will find advertisements for all kinds of so-called pain relievers.

Perhaps the message that I want to leave with you is that your best hope today is to have a group of specialist physicians who can study you carefully from the standpoint of different specialties. So if you have arthritis, chronic headaches, backaches, sciatica, chronic neck pain from whiplash injuries, neuralgias, or pelvic pain, then you will find that in the end your best hope of relief is to cooperate with your doctor, take as small an amount of medication as possible, use whatever physical measures help you, and most of all, develop a positive attitude. *Pain is a fact of life, and no one can escape it.*

I am not as pessimistic as the Spanish philosopher who said: "What is this life that begins amidst the cries of the infant and the screams of the mother?"

Yet, unless we adopt a discipline that life has pain as part of it and there is no pill, gadget, or surgeon's knife that can eradicate it, we are fooling ourselves. Chronic pain is debilitating, wearisome, and has reduced many fine human beings to an almost subhuman level. Sometimes this happens because of drug addiction developing from the well-meaning efforts of a physician who is trying to relieve a patient's pain.

Pain, then, is with us and will stay with us. In the last twenty-five years medical science has made enormous strides in relieving some facets of pain, as I have related here. We can hope for still greater relief in the future. You may be helped within the limits of our medical knowledge today, and you can help yourself to a considerable degree. Herein lies your new hope for relief from pain.

INDEX

173

Miltown, 57
Minnesota Multiphasic Personality Inventory (MMPI), 49–51
Mogul Empire, 32
Morphine, 57, 58
Morton, William Thomas, 17
Mullan, Sean, xii, 164
Myelogram test, 45–47, 52
Myositis, 150
Mystery, Magic and Medicine (Haggerty), 16

National Center of Health, 105
Neal, Patricia, 95, 96
Nerve receptor, 23
Nerve stimulation techniques, 148–149
Nerve surgery, 60–63
Nerve-blocking techniques, 48–49, 59–60
Nerves, cutting (for headache relief), 101–102
Nervous system, 18–26
Nervous tension, importance of avoiding, 126–127
Neuritis and neuralgia, 142–152
  alcohol and, 150–151
  case history, 143–145
  cause of, 110
  of the chest, 149
  and diabetes, 151
  meaning of, 142
  surgery, 148
  treatment for, 146, 151–152
Neurological examination, 40–42
New England Journal of Medicine, 18
Nixon, Richard, 65
Novocain, 7, 18, 49, 54, 146
  for blocking nerves, 59–60
  for headache relief, 100–101
Nucleus pulposus, 108, 113, 120

Occipital neuralagia, 145
Ophthalmoscopic examination, 41–42
Opium, 14

"Pain losers," 69–70
Painful emotions, psychology of, 30–33
Pantopaque, 46, 47
Papanicolaou stain, 158, 161
Parkinson's disease, 64, 85
Pavlov, Ivan, 32, 70
Pelvic pains (in women), 153–158
  doctor's help for, 157
  menstruation, 154–155
  self-help for, 155–156
  simple techniques for relief, 156–157
  surgical treatment, 158
Percodan, 57
Percutaneous cordotomy, xii, 62, 164–165
Peripheral nerves, 23–24
Phantom pain, 29
Phenobarbital, 57
Physical treatments, 58–59
Poliomyelitis, 39
Polysaccharides, 108
Post-Graduate Medicine, 71, 168
Presacral neurectomy, 158
Procaine, 18
Protein, 108
Psychologic techniques, 67–68
Psychologic tests, 49–51
Psychology, 169
Psychosomatic disturbances, 93
Psychosomatic unit, 30
Psychosurgery, 63–65
Pulse diagnosis, Chinese technique of, 66

Quinine, 14, 84